Praise for *Kicking Sick*

"*Kicking Sick* is like the best friend who reminds you of what's possible and holds your hand as you navigate difficulty. This book is brimming with earthy wisdom that will empower your mind and make your spirit shine."

TARA BRACH, PHD
author of *Radical Acceptance* and *True Refuge*

"Amy Kurtz is a highly intuitive resource for practical and inspiring information on how to not only survive with a chronic condition, but thrive. If you have the intention and will to live beyond perceived limits, *Kicking Sick* is a must read for you. Amy can help bring that desire over the finish line."

JOEL M. EVANS, MD
founder and director, The Center
for Functional Medicine

"Amy Kurtz makes it clear that the ultimate jurisdiction for our health destiny is a place within each of us that strives for improvement. Our task is to connect with and ultimately embrace this knowledge. And *Kicking Sick* compassionately guides us to that goal."

DAVID PERLMUTTER, MD
author of the *New York Times* #1 bestseller
*Grain Brain: The Surprising Truth About Wheat,
Carbs, and Sugar—Your Brain's Silent Killers*

"Amy Kurtz shines her brilliant light on the world of chronic illness with humor, honesty, and hope. She creates a practical path filled with wisdom and great advice—showing you that you *can* thrive and you can live an incredible life, no matter what. *Kicking Sick* shows you how."

KRIS CARR
New York Times bestselling author

"Amy is a true leader. With courage and inspiration, she is the ray of light needed to bring awareness to chronic health conditions from the patient perspective, and she coaches you how to embark on the endeavor of you in difficult situations. *Kicking Sick* and Functional Medicine combined are the perfect combination to heal your life."

MARK HYMAN, MD
author of the *New York Times* #1 bestseller
Eat Fat, Get Thin; director, Cleveland
Clinic Center for Functional Medicine

"Amy Kurtz takes the fear out of chronic conditions and replaces it with healing, love, and ease. It takes courage to take the first step toward wellness, but in Amy's hand, the rest of the path is simple to navigate."

TERRI COLE
psychotherapist, coach, and founder
of the Real Love Revolution

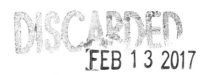

"We all need heroines and happy endings in this rough and tumble world. And we can never get too much inspiration. Amy's book gives us you a healthy dose of all, as you travel with her on her journey to becoming her own healer, reminding you it is possible to go from sick to being a shining Glow Warrior, from hopeless to healthy and happy again. Jump onboard this train for a ride to health freedom."

AVIVA ROMM, MD
director of Thrive Health Center and
author of *The Adrenal Thyroid Revolution*

"Are you among the over 125 million Americans with a chronic illness and are sick of being sick? Then let *Kicking Sick* by Amy Kurtz be your guide to escaping your ineffective disease-management care and reorganizing your approach to escaping illness. Coach Amy will give you a game plan to overcome obstacles and reach your goal of optimum health."

GERARD E. MULLIN, MD
associate professor of medicine, The Johns
Hopkins University School of Medicine;
author of *The Gut Balance Revolution*

"Amy Kurtz in *Kicking Sick* offers an action plan that is not only doable for people who suffer from a chronic condition, it's sympathetic, wise, and courageous. Her tools and strategies get you dealing head-on with yourself, your family, your friends, and your coworkers, and put you back in charge of your own health. Amy not only inspires you, she is you."

LAUREN HANDEL ZANDER
cofounder and chairwoman, Handel Group

"*Kicking Sick* is part of an exciting movement that sees health and well-being as the result of a holistic effort to connect the dots and treat the body as a system, not as separate and unrelated symptoms and problems. Amy Kurtz not only gives personal counsel that is valuable, she brings a series of experts to the table to present a full picture of what great health can look like."

LEO GALLAND, MD,
and JONATHAN GALLAND, JD
international bestselling authors
of *The Allergy Solution*

"If you need a kind, wise friend to help you navigate a chronic illness, Amy Kurtz has written *Kicking Sick* for you. There's a wealth of experience and information here, all aimed at supporting the cultivation of well-being, and shared with a great lightness of spirit."

SHARON SALZBERG
author of the *New York Times*
bestseller *Real Happiness*

"In *Kicking Sick*, Amy Kurtz has deftly consolidated her own practical self-help advice with the wisdom from well-known wellness warriors to help anyone who is chronically ill get out of their *sick* mode . . . If you are looking to break free from the chains of chronic illness, *Kicking Sick* is the book for you. Read every word and take notes!"

VINCENT PEDRE, MD
functional medicine certified practitioner and author of *Happy Gut: The Cleansing Program to Help You Lose Weight, Gain Energy, and Eliminate Pain*

"With love, wisdom, humor, and grace, Amy Kurtz brings chronic conditions out of the shadows, and guides readers on a powerful journey of healing, hope, and renewal. A must-read."

ELENA BROWER
author of *Art of Attention* and *Practice You*

"Amy's book can show you the path to healing your life and your body. When you love your life and body, the message your body receives is filled with live messages. True healing is about more than one's physical self and condition. Read and learn from Amy. All you have to do is show up for practice."

BERNIE SIEGEL, MD
author of *A Book of Miracles* and *Faith, Hope & Healing*

"Amy Kurtz's *Kicking Sick* is a must-read for those trying to navigate the difficult path of chronic illness. Her journey is inspirational and shows that it is possible to rise above and become a better and healthier you."

KEITH BERKOWITZ, MD
medical director, Center for Balanced Health

"Amy Kurtz's inspiring story will motivate readers to take control of their health and heal their bodies. In *Kicking Sick*, she pairs personal experience with key resources that will guide and support anyone who is interested in embarking on their own wellness revolution."

FRANK LIPMAN, MD
author of *10 Reasons You Feel Old and Get Fat*

"Amy Kurtz skillfully guides those with chronic illness on their journey to healing. Knowing yourself holistically, seeking integrative modalities, and actively championing your own wellness are strong remedies for chronic illness and pain."

DEEPAK CHOPRA, MD
author of *Super Genes*

"Amy Kurtz reveals a truth in *Kicking Sick*: the source of wellness is within. Amy inspires us to empower ourselves to elevate and evolve as lead navigator of our own well-being by taking responsibility to learn, love, nourish, and deeply care for our body, mind, and spirit."

PAULETTE COLE
CEO and Creative Director,
ABC Carpet & Home

KICKING SICK

KICKING SICK

your GO-TO GUIDE for thriving
with chronic health conditions

AMY KURTZ

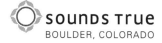
sounds true
BOULDER, COLORADO

Sounds True, Inc.
Boulder, CO 80306

Cover and book design by Rachael Murray

Printed in Canada

Handel Group and *The Handel Method* are registered trademarks of Handel Group.

Library of Congress Cataloging-in-Publication Data
Names: Kurtz, Amy, author.
Title: Kicking sick : your go-to guide for thriving with chronic health conditions / Amy Kurtz.
Description: Boulder, CO : Sounds True, [2017] | Includes bibliographical references.
Identifiers: LCCN 2016022068 (print) | LCCN 2016033038 (ebook) |
   ISBN 9781622036653 (pbk.) | ISBN 9781622037292 (ebook)
Subjects: LCSH: Chronic diseases. | Chronically ill—Care.
Classification: LCC RC108 .K87 2017 (print) | LCC RC108 (ebook) | DDC 616/.044—dc23
LC record available at https://lccn.loc.gov/2016022068

10 9 8 7 6 5 4 3 2 1

For Nina, who showed me that we are so much more than our physical bodies and who taught me that no matter where we are in our health journey, there is always *something* that we can do to improve our quality of life, take care of ourselves better, find light in the dark, and find beauty in the present.

For the one in every two Americans suffering from Chronic Disease, this book is for you.

Contents

Foreword

The disheartening statistic that more than half of Americans are dealing with one or more chronic medical issues personally hit home for me several years ago. I was working between eighty and one hundred hours a week in a busy medical practice, maintaining the exercise routine of a near-professional athlete, and meeting my commitments and obligations as a single father to my two children. In order to fuel this lifestyle, I didn't choose nutritious veggies and wholesome grains or plenty of sleep. Instead, I relied on loads of coffee and sugar to keep me awake and moving.

Not surprisingly, I couldn't sustain this lifestyle. My body broke down, and I developed a severe case of chronic fatigue syndrome. It was a huge wake-up call.

I had to find a way to put myself back together again, and as I tried to do that, I had to confront the fact that the profession I'd dedicated my life to—conventional medicine—couldn't provide all the answers. The body is complex integrated ecosystem, and we have to care for, heal, and nurture the whole system by removing the things that create imbalance and provide the ingredients that create balance. Desperately ill, I went from Harvard to Columbia, saw the best doctors, but none had answers. Then I discovered a new way of thinking about chronic disease based on getting to the root causes and not just focusing on symptoms. The world of Functional Medicine provided a roadmap to health for me and my patients. In fact it is not the science of disease, but the science of creating health. In Functional Medicine we understand that food is medicine, not just calories; it is information that affects every function of your body in real time. Once I understood the power of food to reshape my biology, it was easy to fix my cookies, coffee, and sugar diet. I was eating the wrong foods, and even though I was in great shape, I learned you can't eat poorly and fix it through exercise. I needed Functional Medicine to sort out what could heal me, and it is what connected the dots in Amy Kurtz's healing as well.

Amy's story is very similar to my own. Amy came to me five years ago with thyroid complications, celiac disease, a parasite infection, and a myriad of other health issues that were all affecting each other. She is a perfect example of many of my patients who have tried many traditional ways of healing and haven't yet gotten the care they need. It can be difficult to take a complicated health situation and find the care you need when you have many different doctors giving you different answers that contradict each other. Functional Medicine offers a different paradigm for looking at medicine and achieving health. Given how many issues Amy had from an early age, how many complications evolved, and how many doctors she had saying different things, it would have been easy to feel hopeless. It took a lot of time, energy, and focus for her to take on her health, create a team of people, and create the experience of her illness as a valuable process. I am proud of the amount of deep work she has done in order to heal herself.

Amy took difficulty and pioneered through it. In *Kicking Sick* she shows that there is a better way to heal your life, where you love yourself and you grow from an experience. She has made an amazing case and resource of bringing people together in order to heal others. She used her experience with illness for good. When people go through something hard, many times people make it all about themselves and how hard it is for them. What Amy does so beautifully in *Kicking Sick* is that she pulled all of the cobwebs together and created a beautiful resource for people facing the same challenges that she did. She makes it easy for you to look at it in a new way, one with possibility and hope.

As a doctor and someone who has personally healed through Functional Medicine, the only way I can look at disease is to see the whole body as one integrated system, not a collection of different organs that we separate into medical specialties. I look at the whole person to find the right treatments that address root causes and restore balance in the complex web of our biology that gets people from sick to well. Amy offers the information and the encouragement you need to look at the big picture and see the connections between how you live and how you feel. If you feel you've been sidelined by your illness, this process will help you face how to get into your life with an attitude that makes you choose the endeavor of you. With kindness, humor, and wise advice, you will be ready to take each next best step on your road back to true, vibrant health. *Kicking Sick* is a great place to start your healing!

Wishing you health and happiness,
Mark Hyman, MD

Dear Beautiful You,

I'm so glad and grateful you decided to pick up this book. Thank you. I know what it's like to feel sick, fearful, and isolated because of a chronic health condition. Since 2010 I have been hustling to figure out my health situation, take control of it, have a better quality of life, and not be stuck and desperate for answers. This was not easy, and it took an extraordinary amount of time, but eventually the pieces came together, which allowed me to start feeling better and thrive again. Today, I consider myself lucky to have felt thirty going on eighty. I wrote *Kicking Sick* because I know you can thrive again, too.

Dealing with over a decade of debilitating pain and conditions ranging from celiac disease to a thyroid disorder to a major parasite infection, I embarked on an intense journey through doctors' offices, medical clinics, IV labs, and specialists. The journey was a wake-up call. Did every doctor, healer, specialist, and guru have my best interest in mind? Some did, some didn't. One thing is certain: I made a bucket load of choices that didn't serve me and wasted a good amount of time because of it.

I've now dedicated my life to helping you heal yours and to getting the word out about *Kicking Sick* loud and clear. As a health coach and wellness expert, I am able to relate and deeply connect with clients because I have gone through the struggle myself. I've been where you are. I get it. I know how to simplify the chaotic part of being sick—and figure out how to put human, physical, spiritual, and emotional energies where they belong.

Whether you are currently learning how to navigate a chronic health condition, have recently been diagnosed with a health condition, feel hopeless, or just need some new tips and tricks managing one, *Kicking Sick* is for you.

The turning point in my journey of healing was when I realized how crucial it was to focus on my individual needs and to surround myself with a team of professionals best suited for me. I became an active participant in my own health and got more involved, educated, and invested in the healing process. I started to show up for my own life in a way that I had never done before. I had to learn to love every part of myself again. Everything shifted when I started to see myself as more than my physical condition. Through my shift in energy, focus, and responsibility, I was able to help myself, and I am confident I can help you.

I'm going to give it to you straight. This book was extremely difficult to write because it forced me to relive some of the most painful (physically and emotionally) times of my life. In the depths of dealing with disease in my body, I felt so utterly and completely alone. I felt terrified that my conditions would never improve and that I was destined to be a person who would always struggle with chronic health conditions, feel like an outcast, and suffer from total discomfort in my body. "Sick" leaked out over all of my relationships and onto everything and everyone I touched. I made myself into a helpless victim who stayed a child in many ways—until I decided to choose love over fear, strength over weakness, and independence over dependency.

I am still on my own healing journey, but I have kicked being sick and taught myself how to pick myself up, put one foot in front of the other, and glow in the face of adversity. In doing so, I have become a better patient and a happier person. And I want to show you, my dear friend, how to do the same. I understand how you feel and what you are going through. I did everything wrong so you don't have to.

My prayer is that this book will teach you to become a better friend to your body—to the miraculously intelligent and beautiful vessel that carries your soul through this life. I wrote this book to let you know that you are not alone and to give you the tools you need to thrive through this experience, rather than let it define who you are.

Place your hand on your heart and say, "Even though I'm not perfect, I deeply and profoundly love myself." I'm sending you love too.

From my heart to yours,

Amy

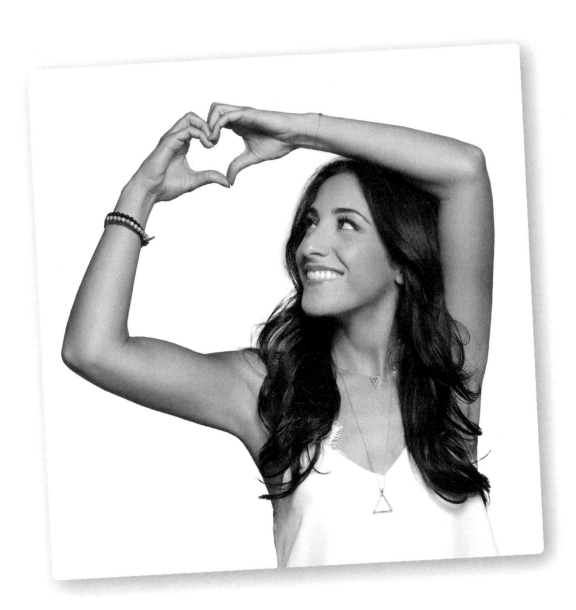

1

What's Amy Got to Do With It?

"Amy!"

"Amy!"

"Amy, honey! Get up, sweetheart. Everything will be okay."

My parents were talking to me, but all I heard were their muffled voices as I lay crumpled on the floor of a prominent specialist's office, tears gushing, my body wracking and shuddering in despair and sadness. The doctor's words echoed in my ears: "Your colon doesn't work; it's totally shot. I have no idea why. You're most likely never going to be able to have a bowel movement on your own ever again. One of the very few options you have is to remove it." Living with a nonfunctioning colon was not part of my life plan. Nor was struggling for five years looking for answers. At first it felt as though my heart had plummeted down a deep, dark, long hole. And then I was numb.

That moment was my rock bottom.

Let me tell you how I got there. I grew up the youngest of three girls in a suburb just outside Philadelphia. My dad is a doctor, my mom is an artist, and there was a lot of love,

laughter, and happy times in our family. I was always on the go, constantly trying to keep up with my older sisters. I was active, playing outside, taking dance classes, singing, swimming, hula hooping, riding my bike, doing arts and crafts, playing pranks on my sister, chasing fireflies in the summertime, and just feeling free. I loved life. I never wanted to miss out on anything.

One night after dance class, I ran upstairs straight to my room. I wanted to do my homework as quickly as possible so I could go back to practicing my dance moves. As I bent down to get my math textbook off the floor, I felt a shooting pain go from the base of my spine all the way up to the top—*clang*, like the disk hitting the bell on a strongman carnival game. I had never felt pain of that caliber before. I couldn't move. Bent over at the waist and frozen that way, I waddled down the hall into my dad's study and cried out, "Daddy, I can't move." He knelt down and held me.

I rested my back for a few days in an attempt to get over the profound spasm. Afterward, I tried to resume my life, but I was never that active, free-spirited, spritely little girl again. I couldn't be. My lower back hurt constantly, and that ran the show from that textbook moment on, for the next eleven years of my life. I tried to dance again, and it hurt too much. I tried to go to field hockey camp with a friend as I had planned, and I couldn't move from the pain I was in. The doctors said, "Don't do it if it hurts," so I stopped doing most of the things I was used to doing freely because of a physical condition that was on the rise, whether I wanted it to be or not.

There was a nerve component to the problem with my back. Basically, it felt as if the nerves in my low back were jumping out of my skin. If I took a walk, I would feel pain. If I played Nintendo with my friends, I would feel pain. If I just sat on the couch, I would feel pain. When I lay in bed at night,

I would feel pain. My body was saying, "Something isn't right here. Pay attention." But I didn't know that. How could I? I was just a child.

As a fourteen-year-old girl with debilitating back pain, I was thrust into a scary adult world of dealing with a chronic illness. I had an illness before I had time to truly have a full childhood. While my friends were going to dance class and playing sports after school, I was going from doctor to doctor, trying to find a solution for the nearly unbearable pain I was in and to understand why I wasn't at home in my body anymore. I was constantly unsettled in my skin. With time, my free spirit and I disconnected.

From the moment I crawled into my dad's home office on all fours, he, my mom, and I were together on a journey. My parents tried

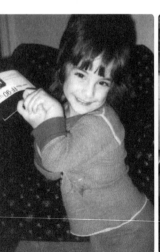 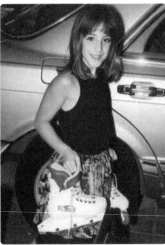 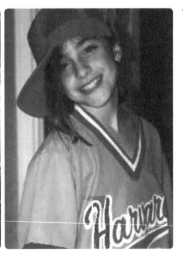

The young me: before my illness, I was an active child who loved life.

the best they could with what they knew. They were with me all the way. This was new for all of us. My dad used all of his resources to get me in to see the best specialists in town. I saw the best of the best. My mother was the schlepper and the nurturer; she was by my side everywhere, holding my hand, kissing me, stroking my hair, keeping me giggling, and supporting me.

We tried everything: physical therapy, back braces, TENS (transcutaneous electrical nerve stimulation) machines, chiropractic care, massage, and the application of ice and heat to the affected areas. None of it worked. It seemed to be a mysterious condition that no one understood. Despite all the treatments and tests, there were no clues as to the root cause of the pain.

Finally, I was put on painkillers three times a day, plus a pill to calm my nerves once a day, and another pill to relax my muscles at night. *When I was fourteen!* These meds were part of my daily routine through middle and high school, and I continued taking them through college. They seemed to work. They numbed the condition—at least for a while. Wasn't taking all those medications the right thing to do because they "worked"? After all, a medical doctor prescribed them. Pain was at the forefront of who I, Amy Kurtz, was. It defined me. I considered it to be "my normal."

But I was also aware that this part of me was different from my friends. I knew that my friends didn't have pain issues. I just thought I was the unfortunate one.

I went to college for a degree in the performing arts and had the dream of being an actor. My body made me feel caged, and acting was the one thing that let me escape

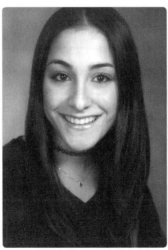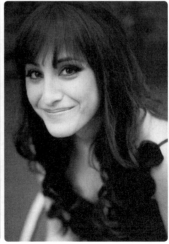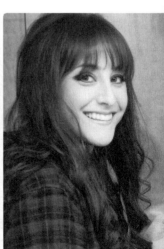

I grew up looking healthy, and no one could tell I wasn't well. From my senior year high school photo (2003) and two photos taken at my sister's wedding (2009), you wouldn't know how much pain I was in or how much medication I was taking to feel "normal."

my reality and express myself freely. I was still always in pain. On top of it, I got the mononucleosis virus my sophomore year. I was so sick I had to move home for the remainder of the semester. I crawled right back into my childhood bed and stayed there until the start of the next semester. Some friends also got mono, but never as severely as I did. I knew it presented itself less severely in them, but I didn't understand why. I never fully recovered from the mono virus, and after that, my back pain kicked me with a new vengeance.

The pain pills had started being less effective as the years went by. Sometime after I got sick with mono, they stopped working entirely. Unless I took even more medication, I would pretty much always have pain. This was devastating because it affected everything—my classwork, my social life, my relationships, my ability to do anything. I was always trying to act like a normal young person, but the reality was I was no such being. Taking heavy-duty pills all the time definitely inspires you to see yourself as sick—and they certainly don't make you feel "better."

The older I got, the more I realized the problem wasn't being fixed by the pills; they were masking a big problem, which was only getting worse. I longed to feel a different way. I longed to no longer feel helpless and physically debilitated. I so wanted to find a way to truly help myself—maybe a healthier lifestyle would make my pain more bearable.

So I decided to show up for my life in a way I hadn't and see if there were any lifestyle changes I could make that might help.

I saw a nutritionist, incorporated whole foods into my diet, and discovered juicing. I ate a lot of veggies and very few processed foods. Essentially, I cut out the crap. Interestingly enough, the changes I made to my diet meant I was mostly eating gluten-free foods. My back pain almost disappeared, and I thought I had discovered the key to the kingdom. It felt great to feel in control and to be able to slowly taper off the medications and move more normally, without constantly being aware of the pain I felt at every moment. All in all, I was doing my version of well. I began planning a move to Los Angeles to pursue my acting goals.

Before I made my big move, I went abroad to Israel. I had fond memories of a trip I had made with my family to my ancestral and spiritual homeland when I was seven. I was

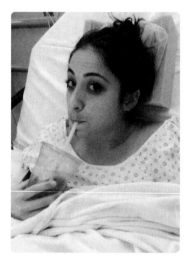

Me in the hospital right after getting back from Israel, after gaining thirty pounds in thirty days.

looking forward to going back as an adult. What began as an exciting adventure to a foreign country ended up as a physical and emotional horror story. I had a total body shutdown during my stay. I was on an organized trip that included a meal plan, and there weren't a lot of healthy food options available. It was slim pickins', and nothing matched the healthy diet I had been eating at home. The offerings included mostly pita bread and hummus. The back pain I had endured my whole life reemerged, times ten. It wasn't just pain this time; my whole body started reacting in a way I had never experienced before—and quickly. When I was seven years old on my first trip to Israel, I climbed the Masada with adults, and I kept up, felt great, and impressed everyone around me with my youthful agility. Now, at twenty-five, I was struggling to keep up with the elderly people on the hike. I looked in front and in back of me and realized

I was the slowest person in the group, lagging way behind everyone. I couldn't catch my breath; I was literally gasping for air, feeling as though I were going to faint.

I gained thirty pounds in thirty days. I had rashes all over my skin; I couldn't keep down any solid food or go to the bathroom. My hair was falling out in clumps, I still couldn't catch my breath, my limbs felt like they were aching off my body, and I had dark black circles under my eyes. My body was completely failing me.

My intention to take a fun trip abroad, come back to the States, and head to the sunny skies of LA and land a speaking part in a movie was busted wide open. Instead, I came back to Philadelphia, walked right back into my childhood bedroom, got under the covers, and sank into total fear, isolation, and desperation.

I was so ill upon my arrival home I could barely muster the strength to stand up and

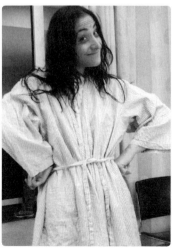

Waiting to have some more tests done. Age 27

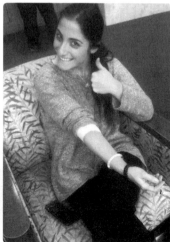

At the Mayo Clinic after my ninth medical test of the day. In good spirits, looking forward to some answers! Age 29

walk. I could not eat anything but liquids: shakes, smoothies, and soups, which, coincidently, were gluten- and dairy-free, so my back pain subsided. Yet I remained so fragile, fatigued, and achy. My hair continued falling out in clumps, I was breaking out in hives as if I were allergic to myself, and I didn't have a bowel movement for an entire month.

During this period, my brain started telling me it was time to go big or go home. I began my quest to find out what was wrong. In addition to my dramatic symptoms came a myriad of diagnoses: a severe parasite infection picked up on my trip abroad, chronic fatigue syndrome, heavy metal poisoning, thyroid disorder, Lyme disease, a slow-transit motility disorder of the colon, small intestinal bacterial overgrowth (SIBO), *and* celiac disease. I was no longer absorbing food or nutrients, I couldn't keep any food down, and I couldn't go to the bathroom. My whole body was in shutdown mode. My gastric system, which had been working so hard for so long and fighting itself at such a deep level, said, "Strike three, you are out!"

I went full speed ahead, in total crisis mode, to seeing everyone and anyone who I thought might have some answers. I went to an assortment of conventional doctors, following all their recommendations to the letter because I was so desperate to get better and get on with my life. I researched every possible cause for my afflictions, like an overzealous junkie on a frantic mission to feed her fix. It was like throwing spaghetti at the wall and seeing what strands would stick. I tried to get better until the point of complete exhaustion—emotionally, physically, and mentally.

Finally, I took a big, long break from all of it, and then I figured out what was real *to me*. Up until this exhausted and extreme state in my life, I was listening to everyone *but me*. It was time for me to start showing up for my own life. It was also time to stop believing that one doctor would have the magic answer and to instead find a reliable, go-to health team. A great deal of research and reading was required to find the right healing path for me. I was very aware that my condition was severe and that I needed to find the correct specialists for my conditions—and quickly. I had grown up thinking that Western medicine was the only kind of medicine that existed. I believe Western medicine is important and has helped me a great deal, but I also wanted to learn about everything else that was out there. I started to explore alternative healing modalities and became interested in the idea of combining many different approaches to healing. I went from one extreme to the next, but I slowly started to figure out a balance, including the healing philosophies that made sense for *me*.

Eventually I found a doctor who correctly diagnosed why I had been plagued with back pain for so many years: celiac disease. In the

1990s, when my pain started, no doctor ever suggested the pain could be food related. Flash forward to the 2000s, and doctors began to realize that gluten and other foods could be the root cause of human disease and disorders. The celiac did not cause every symptom I'd experienced, but it was the cause for my back pain, and it certainly made my body into the perfect host for all the other things that happened to me—including an actual parasite (ew!). Two days after I eliminated gluten from my diet, my back pain was gone forever, as if it had never existed. The pain disappeared just as it had before, when I had inadvertently eliminated gluten from my diet.

I've gone from being a tween in chronic pain to a pill-popping young woman to a woman in charge of her own health and wellness. One thing I learned along the way is that suffering from a chronic health condition should not define who I am. I also learned that I am not alone in my experience. There are so many people out there who, just like me, are dealing with chronic health conditions. One out of every two people in America has at least one.[1]

I didn't get to a place of healing all by myself. I had a lot of help, including medical practitioners and wellness workers who held my hand and were my parachutes throughout my journey. These heroes include Mark Hyman, MD, a functional medicine specialist and founder of the UltraWellness Center and the director of the Cleveland Clinic Center for Functional Medicine; Gerard Mullin, MD, a top gastroenterologist at Johns Hopkins Hospital; Philip Felig, MD, a top endocrinologist; maharishi Thom Knoles; Lauren Handel Zander, cofounder and chair of Handel Group; and others. When I began to think about writing a book for other women with chronic health conditions, I knew that insights from these members of my personal "A-team" would help others as much as they had helped me.

I also knew it was important to include wisdom from my favorite thought leaders—people whose wisdom, philosophy, and approach to life's challenges brought me key "aha moments" and helped me navigate my journey with more grace and ease. These "favorites" include *New York Times* bestselling author and speaker Gabrielle Bernstein; multiple *New York Times* bestselling author, wellness advocate, and cancer thriver Kris Carr; renowned yogi and author Elena Brower; psychologist and fear guru Terri Cole; tapping expert Jessica Ortner; and others.

Finally, I have found a tribe of women who are thriving and succeeding despite the chronic issues they have learned to manage with grace, understanding, and yes, even humor. I call them Glow Warriors: champions of the good life who have kicked the *sick* label, risen above their conditions, and constantly remind me that happiness and healing is possible no matter what my situation. I decided their wisdom and words deserved to be in my book too because it's reassuring to know that, if you have one or more chronic conditions, you're in great company and that all of us, no matter our struggles, can learn to bloom and flourish in so many ways.

Here are the most important things I want you to know: First, you really aren't alone. I know what you are going through, I've felt what you feel, and I've got your back. Second, healing is a journey not a destination, and you need your time, love, and attention. Third, it's time to radically accept where you are at in this exact moment and make the choice to start thriving. And I believe if you're reading this book, you're ready. The time is now.

Let's kick it!

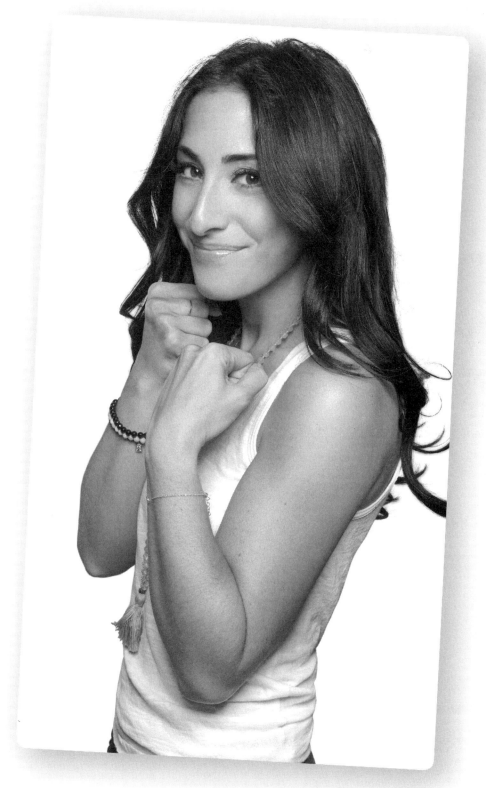

Meet the Glow Warriors

THESE INSPIRING WOMEN remind us that happiness and healing are possible no matter what your situation. These ladies have graciously shared their wisdom throughout the pages of this book.

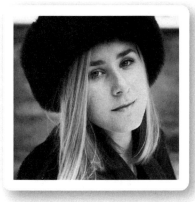

Kaitlyn Lennon

DIAGNOSIS   Polyarticular Rheumatoid Arthritis (RA)

AGE OF DIAGNOSIS   17

OCCUPATION   Client relationship manager by day, artist and crafter by night

OUTLOOK ON HEALING   Be gentle with yourself, both body and mind. Pain is inevitable; suffering is optional.

THE MOST IMPORTANT LESSON I'VE LEARNED FROM MY HEALTH JOURNEY
RA has been one of my greatest teachers, and living with it has had a surprisingly positive impact on my inner growth. It has shaped so much of who I have become, and I am very grateful for the wisdom it has imbued. The need for self-care that comes along with chronic illness has opened me up to practices, people, and experiences that I otherwise would have never pursued. Living with ongoing physical pain also connects us to others in a way that is easy to overlook when things are easy and comfortable. The compassion this inspires is, I feel, one of the most important and precious qualities we can possess and act from as human beings.

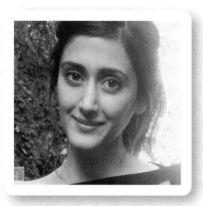

Tara Sowlaty

DIAGNOSIS   Crohn's disease

AGE OF DIAGNOSIS   14

OCCUPATION   Natural foods chef, nutritionist, cofounder of How You Glow

OUTLOOK ON HEALING   Learn the lessons like a pro and break them like an artist. Find the keys to your personal balance of happiness and keep doing those things!

THE MOST IMPORTANT LESSON I'VE LEARNED FROM MY HEALTH JOURNEY Health starts with staying present with your body. When you are in tune with yourself, you will know just what your body needs. We can all be our own healers; we just need some time, patience, and diligence.

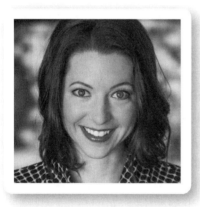

Jennifer Fugo

DIAGNOSES   Gluten, casein, and egg sensitivities; adrenal fatigue; dyshidrotic eczema; hidradenitis suppurativa

AGE OF DIAGNOSES   27

OCCUPATION   Author of *The Savvy Gluten-Free Shopper: How to Eat Healthy Without Breaking the Bank,* health consultant, founder of Gluten Free School

OUTLOOK ON HEALING   Rome wasn't built in a day. All problems are figure-outable; they're just waiting for you to become determined enough to find a solution.

THE MOST IMPORTANT LESSON I'VE LEARNED FROM MY HEALTH JOURNEY There's neither a quick fix nor a magic bullet. Beware of fad diets and assuming that someone else's solution will be your own. Healing takes time and often involves uncovering many layers of ill health before you find answers.

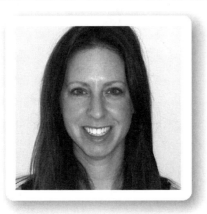

Morgan Segal

DIAGNOSIS Erythromelalgia

AGE OF DIAGNOSIS 27

OCCUPATION High school special education teacher

OUTLOOK ON HEALING I am strong; I will get through this.

THE MOST IMPORTANT LESSON I'VE LEARNED FROM MY HEALTH JOURNEY
Pain is pain. Everyone has it in some way, though the definition and feeling of pain is different for everyone. I have more patience and a greater appreciation for life. I can get through anything because I am strong, and I am very lucky to have learned this on such a profound level!

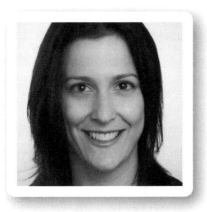

Lindsay White

DIAGNOSIS Remitting and relapsing multiple sclerosis

AGE OF DIAGNOSIS 28

OCCUPATION Advertising executive

OUTLOOK ON HEALING Everyone has something; it is what you do about it and how you handle it that matters.

THE MOST IMPORTANT LESSON I'VE LEARNED FROM MY HEALTH JOURNEY
I appreciate how lucky I am and that there is always someone who has it worse. Live in the moment, enjoy life, and don't let yourself get sucked into the vortex of negativity and fear. The future will bring what it will, and I know I will deal with it as it comes.

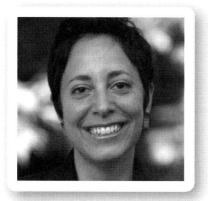

Paige Marmer

DIAGNOSIS Breast cancer (stage 2A)

AGE AT DIAGNOSIS 33

OCCUPATION Psychologist

OUTLOOK ON HEALING Find support, support, support. Allow people in and give yourself permission to be vulnerable. Allow yourself to cry, to grieve all that you will lose from the diagnosis. I hate that I have no sensation left in my breasts, but for me, it's important to focus on what I gained. And I gained so much: perspective, true love for myself, patience, appreciation for the value of imperfection, and so many other countless things. My diagnosis brought me closer to myself and others.

THE MOST IMPORTANT LESSON I'VE LEARNED FROM MY HEALTH JOURNEY
Life is short; live it. That sounds so cheesy and cliché, but for me, it's so true. Since recovering from cancer, I have embraced life in a way that I never thought possible. I have created a new life for myself, a new comfort level that has come from putting myself out there and receiving so much back. I'm *so* grateful for where I've ended up. I'm not sure I'd be so happy in my life now if it weren't for going through the cancer journey. I will never refer to it as a bad experience. Because it wasn't—it gave me so much more than it took away. I'm grateful that I had it. I know that it sounds so fucking crazy, but it's true.

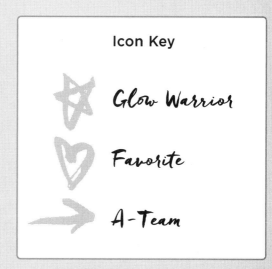

Icon Key

☆ *Glow Warrior*

♡ *Favorite*

→ *A-Team*

2

From Sick Chick to Glow Warrior

In my senior year at college I was involved in a school tradition called "Marathon," where every freshman was assigned to a senior, and that freshman makes fun of you in a series of theater skits. My freshman's performance was eye-opening. She whined, "I can't do this, and I can't do that. My neck hurts, my back hurts, my shoulders ache." Everyone in the audience was laughing, but I was hurt and surprised. *That's* how my classmates saw me? As a whiner and a complainer—a joke? A hypochondriac? Everyone else's skit portrayed something truly funny, but I had a real health problem. And I was being laughed at for it.

There's a reason why chronic illnesses are considered the "invisible diseases" and sometimes perceived as hypochondria: if others actually can't *see* the pain you're in, they think you're a faker. The truth is, I actually *did* think of myself as a "sick chick" for a long time, so I bear responsibility for transmitting that message out to the masses.

Feeling truly ill after I came back from Israel, I naturally went right back to projecting the sick chick persona I was apparently famous for. It's understandable. And that's the irony: until we stop defining ourselves as sick, other people will continue to see us that way too.

I am not my body; my body is the house that holds my soul. It took a long time for me to learn this. It's a major transition in thinking we must make when we have a chronic condition or *dis*-ease in our body, at least if we want to have a chance of living a whole, happy, radiant life. We have to take very good care of that shell and keep searching for the right treatments, but we do have "bad days." Everyone with a chronic illness knows what I'm talking about: the days when we just want to pop out of our bodies and into some other perfect body, one with no colon problems, stomach issues,

> *I am not my body; my body is the house that holds my soul.*

no backaches, headaches, wheezing, or itchy rashes. I get it.

What I didn't realize for a long time, back when I saw myself as a sick chick, is that my body *is* perfect, even on those inevitable bad days. Although having a chronic condition can be absolutely horrible, the experience of having chronic conditions can also be a great gift. No, I'm not kidding. The side effects are astounding. I frequently hear the same idea from other women who have chronic health issues: "I didn't know who I was before I had a chronic issue to deal with." A chronic illness really does redefine priorities, purpose, and happiness. Hell, it even redefines your ideas of what fun and friends are. I have become more present, compassionate, patient, tenacious, and loving. When I was really sick and my body was seriously failing, my purpose, passions, and love of life became crystal clear. What matters and what does not matter, who deserves my energy and who doesn't—it all became obvious. Too many of us never get around to making

> *You are not your sickness, and defining yourself that way means you will be sick for the rest of your life.*

Kick "Sick"

I don't even want you to use the word *sick* anymore. That word is so small. And you are so expansive. Write *sick* on a piece of paper, and take it to your kitchen sink. Crumple it up in a ball, light a match, and burn that paper to ashes. Then rinse out the sink and let the remains float down the drain. Give that word a swift kick in the ass! Sayonara, sweetheart! You are bigger than that word; it will not and cannot defeat you anymore.

and setting priorities and boundaries. But those of us with chronic issues have to set limits and make top-ten lists.

So listen up: you are *not* your sickness, and defining yourself that way means you will be sick for the rest of your life. There is no way I'm going to let you live the life of a sick person. You are not in a healing crisis; you are being offered a healing opportunity; it is time to seize it! Instead of viewing your condition as a dis-ease in your body, choose to view it as an opportunity to reconnect with yourself and learn to love yourself. You are a beautifully strong, shining, resilient Glow Warrior.

Redefine Yourself: Connect with Your Soul

We get down and dirty about the squishy, God-Universe-Gaia-Bliss stuff in chapter 8, but I need to touch on it for a moment here since making friends with your inner self—your real self—is important when it comes to seeing yourself as a person who lives well. When I discovered the Glow Warrior within, I knew it definitely came directly from the power of the Universe (you can call it God, the One, or Gaia—it all works; let's not get stuck on semantics). It's there within you too—you just gotta reach in and grab it. Don't worry—you'll never go *too* far in. You won't drown, get lost, or lose your way. You will, however, start seeing yourself as bigger than your physical challenges or limitations.

Do Nothing—with Purpose

First of all, don't just sit there. Sit there and get comfortable in the *present moment.* The first step to truly healing is to fully surrender to where you are in this moment. And to let it be. When you allow yourself to be truly present in your body, your heart will soften and open, and you can begin to use that feeling as your guide. This is how you will begin to heal yourself. Focusing on your breath is what will bring you back to the present at any moment you choose. Your breath is your life force and your anchor, and unfortunately it is something that, for a lot of us, tends to get lost in the

Don't just sit there. Sit there and get comfortable in the present moment.

shuffle when we are dealing with severe stress in the body. The first place to start getting reconnected to yourself is through your breath.

Focus on breathing in through your nose, lowering your breath all the way down into your tummy, and expanding your ribcage out to the sides. Then slowly exhale out through your mouth. The first time I sat and did nothing but breathe, I thought I was going to scream hard enough to ace the part of the hysterical heroine in the next zombie apocalypse movie. After a few tries I started looking forward to it because doing nothing *with purpose* really does put you in touch with your higher self, your inner guide, the present moment, and the spiritual forces that are all on your side. It's called meditating, which is a practice that helps us build and maintain our internal energy and develop patience, forgiveness, and compassion.

If you have a chronic condition or are physically struggling, you have to make a clear intention to sit in the initial discomfort and distractions beginning meditation often brings. There you are, sitting cross-legged, replaying a particularly annoying

Simple Meditative Breathing

Sit still and tall somewhere comfortable; a chair with good back support works well. Close your eyes and begin breathing through your nose. Inhale for a count of two, and exhale gently for a count of four. Keep breathing evenly and smoothly. Set a timer and breathe this way for at least five minutes.

One nice element you can add to this exercise is a mantra. On the inhale say to yourself, "I am," and on the exhale, say to yourself, "perfectly well." In doing so, you're tuning into the idea that you're not just your physical ailments, and you're making room for your true self to breathe. Afterward you will notice a positive difference in your mood.

conversation at work, or thinking about the laundry you need to pick up (or dry cleaning you need to drop off), and all of a sudden you're not meditating anymore. Eventually, you re-center yourself and let those random thoughts float by (bye-bye!), and you do begin to see yourself differently. You begin to feel more loving and more forgiving, less critical of yourself. You get yourself out of the "what ifs" of the future or "coulda shouldas" from the past and get comfortable in the present moment.

Don't stop even if you feel very uncomfortable and strange in the beginning. Be persistent. Give time and space for your inner voice to make itself heard. That will happen either right in the moment or sometime later during the day. Doing nothing is so powerful it has an amazing residual effect—sort of like taking a time-release capsule of inner peace and wisdom. Some synchronistic event will occur; someone will tell you exactly what you need to hear; you will get a sudden flash of insight. Along with that, you'll realize you are so much more than your tingling legs, irritable bowel, or migraine headache.

Stop thinking about the piece of cheese you weren't supposed to eat yesterday or the IV you need tomorrow. As Ram Dass says, "Be here now," *right now*. Look, I can still be meditating and repeating my mantra and suddenly Beyoncé will pop into my head. I just shake it out—sorry, B! Or I make it work, and I say a mantra (see page 125) to the beat of the song. Just roll with it. But most importantly, be with yourself, in stillness, and breathe. You can tap into who you really are underneath the truckload of emotional crap you are carrying around just by giving yourself this space to breathe and connect with your heart. When you connect with your inner guide and get in touch with your heart, you can change your thought process at any moment.

Connect with Your Inner Glow Warrior

Have a dialogue with your inner Glow Warrior and your heart. For the next twenty-one days (that's long enough to create a habit), stay in touch with her throughout the day: "Hey, Glow Warrior, I know you're there, and I want to get to know you and hear what you have to tell me. I want to listen to your wisdom. Give me a head's up. Show me how to connect with you and how to show up for it." If you're at work, you might want to do this silently, to yourself. But if you're home alone, let her rip—and say it right out loud if it feels right. Eventually, your inner Glow Warrior will start speaking to you in many ways—through clearer insights, more compassionate thinking, and subtle messages you receive at seemingly random times. Don't get frustrated if it seems like a one-way conversation for the first few days or even a week or more. You may have been out of touch with your spirit for years, so it takes a while to dust things off and get the connection going again.

When you become angry with your chronic health condition—and hell yeah, it happens—don't let it get the better of you. Instead, when you feel angry, look inside yourself, practice the breathing, and connect back to your heart. There have been moments when I haven't been thrilled about rescheduling things to accommodate my condition, but I accept it and rearrange it with ease because I want to stay healthy. I look at my old feelings of anger and frustration in a new way now, one that takes me out of sick chick mode and into Glow Warrior power mode. To paraphrase what the great spiritual teacher Thich Nhat Hanh said in his book *Anger: Wisdom for Cooling the Flames,* care for your anger, because anger is an energy that makes us and the people around us suffer. To alleviate overwhelming feelings of anger, do breathing exercises, or if you can, a body scan (see page 38). Ask your Glow Warrior for some help along with the Universe. Smile at your anger—and tell her you love her anyway.

Put an End to Useless Worry

I come from a long, proud line of worriers. One of the things that can prevent us from moving beyond our chronic conditions—aside from the very obvious effects of symptoms (we'll work on those too later in the book)—is *worrying* about the symptoms. I could literally find a way to worry about something all day long, in every possible way. Worry has been a very real part of my being since my back pain started. I have to make a very conscious effort *not* to worry, and getting stuck on the worry train in the past has been overwhelming at times. I have to check myself before I wreck myself, on a pretty consistent basis, and laugh at the worrier who wants to peek out her head and yap at me.

People with chronic conditions worry a lot, but worrying puts us in stress mode and only fear-induced thoughts come out of it. Worry keeps us in our sick mode. Someone said worrying is like praying for a future you don't want. It takes us away from the right now and prevents us from living in the present moment.

Whenever you have a worry or a question that is related to a worry, write it down on a piece of paper and stick it in a box you designate as your Worry Later Box. That way, you can acknowledge the worry, purge it out onto paper, see it in writing, but then file it for another day you can devote to worrying. Now, I don't know how *you* will handle this, but so far I have yet to devote a single day to my Worry Later Box. Worrying isn't a particularly productive action. And because it causes worry lines on your brow, it's also not so cute! So save on your future Botox bills and put those worries away. By making a note of random worries and filing them away, I acknowledge them, and I don't have to spend any more time on them. I can focus on more important things, like spending time with friends, creating a great meal, reading a good book, seeing a movie—all sorts of things that worry prevents.

There's no hocus-pocus here. These practices really do get you out of your I-am-just-my-body mode and into the I-am-so-much-more-than-just-my-body mindset. This is what makes the difference between sick people and well people who happen to also have a chronic condition.

Live Life Beyond Doctors' Offices

Living with a chronic condition can mean lots of trips to the doctor or many trips to many different kinds of doctors if you have a cocktail of chronic conditions or have a condition that has not been diagnosed properly or completely. Sitting around in doctors' offices is a bitch. It can also, quite naturally, turn you into a sick chick if you are not careful. Because believe me, doctors' offices are full of sick chicks. A lot of them are so into their role that they compete for the title of Queen of the Sick Chicks. You do not want to be that girl. Believe me, you don't want a gold medal in illness. It's not worth it, and the endorsement deals suck.

My approach to getting away from the *sick chick* label even when you're on a first-name basis with every lab technician within thirty miles of your house is this: go to doctor's

Worry keeps us in our sick mode.

If you have to be at the doctor's often, don't make it your life. Instead, bring your life to the doctor's office.

appointments, do what you need to do there, and live your life in between. A doctor's appointment is something you must attend to as part of your health regime, just like eating well, exercising, and sleeping. For a person with chronic issues, going to the doctor is just part of the routine, and that's the way it should be.

When you meet a sick chick in the waiting room, send her lots of telepathic love. You can even chat her up, but don't play the I'm-so-sick-my-insurance-company-named-a-plan-after-me game with her. Both of you always lose.

There was a time I was getting daily vitamin shots and vitamin-mineral IVs, going through chelation for heavy metals, and so on, so I have spent a lot of time in this dynamic. I could have moved into the doc's office I was there so often. I didn't just go and leave; I got all up in it. I became friendly with the staff, made friends with the other patients, and lived there, essentially.

So trust me, if you have to be at the doctor's often, don't make it your life. Instead, bring *your life* to the doctor's office. Answer

emails, bring a great book, make yourself an empowering playlist, bring cozy socks or a warm blanket that you love, snuggle up with your fave TV show on your iPad, or bring a journal and write your dream for how you would love to feel in a month, a year, and so on. Ask a friend to come and kick it with you. Stay in *your* zone. It may feel weird at first, but just making the conscious choice to bring in the things that make you *you* will make you feel better while you are there.

Aim for Compassion, Not Perfection

In your quest to live well, you are not becoming a perfect person. That idea implies there's something wrong with you now, and that's simply not the case, my sweets. We aren't meant to be perfect. We are meant to be whole. You are human. It is in our DNA to make mistakes, to be beautifully less than perfect, to fail, to do and say things we wish we hadn't. Luckily, there's tomorrow and the next day, so you can try again. In fact, at any moment you can choose to start again. Give yourself credit where credit is due.

This is the incredible gift of self-compassion: to see ourselves with clarity, diagnosis and all; to understand more deeply our emotions, reactions, and struggles; to wrap ourselves in the arms of our own loving support; and to be comforted and inspired and accepted. It is

You have the ability to heal yourself.

a gift no one can give you or take away from you. It's all about you, baby. It is the fertile ground from which a more compassionate world arises. Everything we experience is, first and foremost, a personal experience, filtered through the lens of our own inner terrain. Compassion for each other flows naturally from the springs of compassion we nurture for ourselves.

You Are Your Own Best Healer

On my journey I have met several earth angels who have skills and knowledge to help me heal. One sparkly healer, a colon therapist with long, wavy hair, essential oils everywhere, and a grounded and authentic presence, was truly present with me in a way I hadn't experienced before. I felt seen, heard, and safe with her. She made me feel taken care of.

In the throw-spaghetti-at-the-wall-and-see-what-sticks state I was in, I would bring a bucket load of new questions about doctors and treatments to every session with her. I'd frantically ask her about this and that treatment, option, fix, or idea. I was looking for instant results and was desperate to find a cure instead of experiencing and connecting to my ailments, loving them, and choosing to heal them with intention. Over the course of our work together, she would always look right into my eyes and tell me, "You have the ability to heal yourself." At first, the three amigos—my ego, judgment, and I—thought, *yeah right, that's easy for you to say.* But she would repeat it every single time I saw her. *Every single time:* "You have the ability to heal yourself." I felt the truth of her words in my soul.

A year later my sparkly healer's practice closed abruptly, and I felt that I would literally not be able to survive without her or the work we were doing to heal my digestive system. In reality, she had been laying the groundwork for my success. Since she had shut down her business and moved to a new area, I had no choice but to trust my instincts. It was in that moment that I realized no one else could take control of and heal my situation but me. She was right: I was and am my own best healer. Going forward, I could meet people who would lovingly care and take the time to help me, but I would never fully heal my life unless I started to truly love myself.

Saying those words, "You have the ability to heal yourself," to myself became my *own* ritual. Those words are part of my daily meditations, and they are now in my bones, a deep knowing. *You* have the ability to heal yourself. I have the ability to heal myself: that lesson became my life.

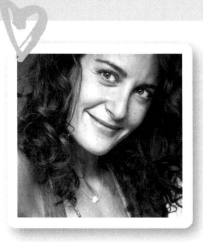

Elena Brower

Elena Brower is the author of *Art of Attention,* a renowned yoga workbook, now translated into five languages. Studying and teaching since 1998, she's respected globally for her distinct blend of alignment and attention in her teaching of yoga and meditation. Her audio meditation coursework, *Cultivating Spiritual Intelligence,* is beloved for its accessibility and relevance, and her yoga teaching is influenced by several traditions, including Katonah Yoga, Kundalini Yoga, and ParaYoga. Elena is also the founder of Teach.yoga, a global website for teachers, and her second book, *Practice You,* will be published in 2017 by Sounds True. Practices with Elena can be found on the website YogaGlo.

For Elena, yoga and meditation have been pathways bringing her back home to her body, to herself, and to love. Her words here are an inspiration to all of us yearning to love ourselves into wholeness.

Welcome. You're here to heal yourself. You're here to traverse the terrain from pain to recovery, from hurt to healing, from confusion to clarity.

You're here to experience love—for yourself.

For decades of my life, I felt disconnected from pleasure, from feeling well, from trusting in myself. As a result, I couldn't connect to the world, I never felt whole, and I couldn't trust others. I became an addict, swimming in self-hatred, and couldn't imagine loving myself. Ever.

To begin finding my way on this path, I began practicing yoga, which had one crucial result: it helped me start *listening.* Before yoga, I couldn't listen to my own body, I couldn't speak its language, and I certainly hadn't ever taken the time to hear or respect its signals. Once I began listening to the profound longing for wholeness inside, I began exploring what might help answer the call I was hearing from deep within me. I realized I was mercifully being called home. ▸

How does yoga work? It places us into moments of undivided attention on our breathing, our architecture, and our physiology, so we can begin to enter into a relationship with our body that transcends thought. It's simply physical, at least initially. Ultimately, it calls us home into a relationship with ourselves that becomes both the physical and the emotional foundation for how we approach everything.

Meditation helped me refine my listening and taught me to learn how to be more sensitive—both to content and context. Meditation helped me recover from my addictions. Meditation helped me remember that my love is wise and it's for me first. Then it taught me that once I can love myself, I have the capacity to extend my highest love to my family, my tribe, my colleagues.

How does meditation work? It gives us periods of time where we can enter into a quiet, effortless period of releasing. For those minutes each day, my body has the time to release doubt, fear, drama, pain, and chaos. Once those are released, I can cooperate with my highest learnings, my finest understandings, and my dreamiest inspirations.

There's been one crucial understanding gained from meditation. When I notice a resistance arising, a judgment crossing my field, I now know that it's just a little pocket of my own internal doubt departing from my body and from my life.

Now, whether I'm practicing yoga or meditation, I'm practicing willingness—to listen, to note, to watch, to let go. Willingness to celebrate and honor the mystery of this existence with all its trials and victories.

How do we stay willing to grow, especially in light of a chronic health condition? Watch and notice. Listen well. Be ready to practice releasing beliefs, doubts, pains, fears—and to welcome in a brand new love that changes everything. ∎

3

Self-Care Is Health Care

We are living in an age where our lives are spinning out of control. We're expected to immediately answer texts and emails; we're constantly faced with new food, entertainment, and information choices; we have to make sure we take care of our needs—all on top of managing our chronic health condition. This overload usually means something falls off the wagon. Unfortunately, more often than not self-care is the *only* activity that makes it possible for us to manage all the demands placed on us. If you had said *self-care* to me in 2010, I wouldn't have known what you were talking about. Today self-care is my basis for living well.

What Is Self-Care, Anyway?

Self-care just sounds really nice, doesn't it? You've probably heard people refer to the idea—as in, "I need to take better care of myself," or "I'm going to be good to myself this weekend." Still, in my experience, a lot us are fuzzy on what self-care is and how to make it part of our routine. Frankly, I never

even knew self-care was a "thing" before Kris Carr made me aware of it through her books. Apparently, self-care has been around for a long time—I just didn't know it.

> *Self-care is not self-indulgence or avoiding healthful choices in favor of quick and short-lived fixes.*

Many of us equate self-care with treating ourselves to things that may actually decrease our well-being. I often hear women say they are going to "take good care of themselves" by meeting their girlfriends at a wine bar, picking up a double-shot latte with extra cream and double raw sugar, or doing some retail therapy and buying a pair of expensive boots they really can't afford. Let's break that habit and rethink the idea of rewards. Self-care is not self-indulgence or avoiding healthful choices in favor of quick and short-lived fixes.

If we don't create ways to disconnect from the world and give ourselves room to breathe, rest, and reflect, we're screwed. One of the first things we learn to do as kids is self-soothe, but as we grow older in a world filled with convenient distractions, we may forget this very important survival skill. I definitely lost my ability to self-soothe the minute my pain started and my spunky free spirit and I disconnected. My frantic search for answers and help had me racing so fast that I had no time to think about what I actually needed.

My sweet mom saw what was happening to me and observed it for a while. One day she said to me softly, in the way only a mother can, "Amy, maybe you need to cry." My initial reaction was to jolt. "Huh? How can I cry?

Self-care is always being there for ourselves, treating ourselves like we would someone we love, and making choices that increase our long-term emotional and physical health and sense of well-being.

I'm so busy! I have to get better!" That pivotal doc appointment, when I was crying on my knees, was the moment, three years after the onset of symptoms, I finally let myself go. I cried and then cried some more. I cried for three days. I cried for the pain I had felt, I cried for the emotional pain that was on my shoulders through the experience, and I cried for my body. I cried for all of it.

When the waterfall finally stopped, it felt divine. I felt present. It felt like I was wrapping myself in my arms, giving myself a big, warm, thoughtful hug. The moment was profound. I felt held by myself. And I thought to myself, what else could I do to make myself feel this good?

I learned that self-care is a way of practicing self-soothing techniques so they pay dividends when it comes to the rest of your life. It's a way of making yourself feel safe and protected because it's when you feel safe that you can truly begin to heal. I went through twenty years of my life with no mechanism for stress reduction. I didn't even realize that quality of life was a "thing" before I stopped speeding like a cokehead jacked up on fight-or-flight adrenaline.

Self-care is always being there for ourselves, treating ourselves like we would someone we love, and making choices that increase our long-term emotional and physical health and sense of well-being, like choosing to exercise, eating healthy foods, getting enough sleep, practicing relaxation techniques, spending time in nature, taking long walks, and engaging in and enjoying a variety of creative pursuits. It begins by creating the space for you to take care of *you*. In short, self-care is everything that this book is about.

Research shows that people who neglect to nurture themselves are in danger of deeper levels of unhappiness, low self-esteem, poor overall health outcomes, and feelings of fear, anxiety, and resentment. Women who spend their time only taking care of others are at risk for depression, burn out, and low energy. We need to emphasize taking care of ourselves *first*. Self-care and stress reduction are mandatory when we are going through the process of healing a chronic health condition. Our bodies need extra TLC, and so does every other part of us. It is mandatory for loving ourselves into wholeness.

Start to incorporate things you truly love into your life. Stay active by doing things that are important to you: pursue a hobby (gardening, painting, crafts—whatever engages you), get involved in your local community, see friends and family you truly love (not the ones who irk you), do work that gives you a sense of purpose and fulfillment. Self-care includes looking at what you *can* do and *want* to do, rather than what you can't do or dislike doing. It means doing things that make you feel good, that make you feel yummy and *better* than you were before you did them.

> "You have to believe that your health challenge happened for a reason. Life is not out to get you; we're not here to suffer. The body is an amazing creation, and it wants to support you. But when you live out of alignment with what your body needs to feel good, it can have problems keeping up."
>
> *Jennifer Fugo*

Are you in the right place, and if not, where do you need to be to get to that feeling? Go there. Because it's all about you, baby. The greatest relationship you will ever have in this life is the relationship you have with yourself. Build it. Strengthen it. Tend and maintain your belief in your own strength, grace, and awesomeness.

Feel the Luv!

The most important thing you can do for your entire being is love it. I know: when you are physically struggling with a chronic condition, love is often the first emotion to be abandoned. I had moments where I hated my body; I was so angry at it for letting me down and not working the way it was "supposed to." I was full of rage toward it. I despised it. I wished that I could hop out of my own busted, swollen system and hop right into another person's active, young, and fully functioning bod so I could live the life I had dreamed of.

Give Yourself a Mirror Moment

Get yourself a fairy godmother mirror, or designate one you already have by sprinkling it with some fairy dust.

Now look in that mirror. Right now. I don't care if your face is puffy or you're wearing granny panties. The more raw you feel, the better, at least for what you're about to do.

Look in that mirror *hard,* but with ease. Truly take yourself in. Take a couple long deep breaths, and give me one thing you love about yourself, physically, spiritually, emotionally, or intellectually. Something truly groovy and amazing about who you are: "I love the freckle above my lip," or "I've got great boobs," or "I'm an extremely good baker. My gluten-free carob-walnut brownies rock." "My arms look extra toned and cut today." "I love my beauty mark. It gives me character." "I love the color of my eyes." "I love my kind heart." "I'm smart and can beat my boyfriend at Scrabble, but I'm also generous and kind, so I let him win every once in a while too."

Now give me something else. Come on, say it out loud. Discover how incredible you are, right now, in this very moment. By doing this, you are committing to being compassionate toward yourself. You are fully taking in your true essence, not your illness. When we give ourselves these moments repeatedly over time, it creates a ritual of self-love. You can then start to have a loving dialogue with yourself, and get on your team. Full acceptance of yourself is the first true step toward healing.

The truth is, I was very angry with my body for a very long time. "Why is this happening to me? Why aren't you working? You piece of crap. How could you do this to me? How could you let me down?" This is how I talked to myself and about myself. It was as if my body were an entity other than me, as if there were two of me next to each other on a bench, and one of us did not care for the other. I didn't say it out loud, but boy did I feel it. That self-talk and all of those feelings resonated through my entire being, all of my physical systems, and every pore and out into every relationship.

Self-care starts with loving yourself—every part of you. Whether you have an annoying zit or a much more serious problem, commit to loving it. Brené Brown says, "Talk to yourself like you would to someone you love."[1] This starts with new, simple, and positive thoughts. Whether small or large, all of our thoughts affect our reality—and you have control over your thoughts. Which means new, positive thoughts can change your reality. When you see a zit on your face and that negative thought comes by *(Ugly! Disaster! I'm hideous!),* say, "I love this zit. This is my zit, and I live for it and love it." The first step toward taking care of yourself well is starting to catch the negative thoughts and being honest and truthful about them. Then you can begin to replace that self-hate thought with a self-loving one.

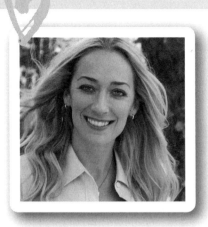

Kris Carr

Kris Carr is the ultimate Glow Warrior and my personal hero. She's been thriving and living with an incurable yet slow-growing cancer since her diagnosis in 2003, and in that time she has made a commitment to learning and sharing what she knows about living well with a chronic condition. Even though her cancer can't be cured, she knows she can still be healthy, and an active participant in her own well-being. Kris hit the road on a self-care journey. Along the way she has written and produced five books, including *New York Times* bestsellers and an award-winning film, *Crazy Sexy Cancer.*

Here, Kris lets us all know how we can truly and deeply care for ourselves.

For me, self-care is simple. It is about being a kind friend to myself. It is listening to my needs, tending my wounds, creating boundaries so I don't get exhausted, fueling my body instead of draining it, and practicing the art of loving all parts of me, from my toes to my tummy, my hair and my nails.

Self-care is also a mindset. It means that we believe we matter. One of the biggest obstacles to self-care is forgetting ourselves in the fog of friends, commitments, deadlines, and demands. You can eat organic food all day and practice yoga consistently, but if you're stressed and angry (at yourself, your friends, your life), much of the goodness goes to waste.

Self-care doesn't have to be all or nothing, and it certainly doesn't have to be perfect. It just needs to work for you. So I've got a five-step plan that should get you started.

1 SELF-CARE REQUIRES A ZERO-NEGATIVITY POLICY. *You* set the tone. Just doing one thing for yourself each day is a positive step in the right direction. I continuously explore how to feel great and how to make a difference. When we feel good and take care of ourselves, we bring that energy and positivity to everything we do. Our relationships improve, our work life gets better, and doors that were previously closed begin to open. Put your soul into self-care, and wrap it in love. When you share ▶

your stories from a vulnerable space, people feel it and let it in.

2   IF YOU'RE SERIOUS ABOUT SELF-CARE, YOUR FAVORITE WORD SHOULD BE *NO.* Saying no is often a very big *yes* for yourself. Yay, you! We all have jobs, families, friends, treatments, doc appointments—the works. You have to be realistic about how much energy you really have available for others and for yourself. My litmus test, when someone asks me to do something, is to ask myself how I feel about it. If it's not a "hell yeah!" it's a "heck no." If I am not feeling it, why am I doing it?

Of course we all have obligations, but I am amazed when I look at my schedule and see so many things I agreed to do, but didn't actually have to do or want to do. These are things that have nothing to do with what my heart is telling me. I am not a yes Pez dispenser. Neither are you. Get really clear on your priorities and know not all of them can happen in one season, or even in one year. The opportunities don't dry up when you say no to others and you say yes to yourself! We're skittish about saying no because we're afraid we'll miss out or people will forget about us, but that's simply not true. Just take a deep breath because there is another train following the one that just left the station. If you fixate on the one you missed, you'll overlook the new one coming down the tracks. When you're doing what you're supposed to do, doors open.

3   GIVE YOURSELF THE GIFT OF SELF-KNOWLEDGE. You already know what you like and what you don't like. If you don't know how you feel, you have too much going on. If you can't tap into your emotions, you're spread too thin. Stop. Breathe. Look at what you're doing, and remove from your plate the things that don't make you happy. Scrape them right off into the trash bin. Learn to surrender, and go to a deeper level of befriending yourself. The more you allow that knowledge to speak to you, the easier life becomes. People who are resilient are in touch with their inner voice and, as a result, create the energetic reserve they need. You don't need to ask anyone for permission or approval. You have all the answers. Instead of running to the latest workshop or guru, you need to slow down and tap into your gut wisdom. My gut never leads me astray.

4 FIND YOUR HAPPINESS WITH BABY STEPS. Happiness is not a fixed state. You don't achieve it and put it in a backpack. Happiness is a direction you are or should always be moving toward. Happiness can simply be feeling content on the journey. What made me happy at nineteen is very different from what makes me happy now. So don't expect your happiness to be the same as it used to be. Think about what makes you happy right now. Start small. Does it make it you happy to pet your dog? Do that. Does it make you happy to take a walk or visit with a certain person? Do that. Replace the things you don't like with the people and activities that truly fill you with joy. Take little tiny bites to start, and get the flavor of doing things you love, for you. That feeling may be a stranger to you, but getting to know it again is essential.

5 GO WHERE YOU NEED TO BE. If you have no space for creativity, you cannot create health or whatever it is that you're here to create. For me, getting where I needed to be meant getting out of New York City. I'd moved to Manhattan at nineteen and had a fun, crazy life. When I had to deal with my forever stage-4 cancer diagnosis, I needed to do that in the mountains. I still love to visit New York, but after three days, we have to part ways. I need to be near nature and near animals and to realign myself with different core values than those I was familiar with in New York.

Everyone has her own journey. For me, seeing that I was not cancer was key. This is especially important since I am living with an untreatable cancer; it would be so easy to identify as a cancer patient. But truthfully, I am only a cancer patient when I go to the doctor a couple of times a year. I want to create a rich life and learn what the diagnosis teaches me, which is neither denial nor defining myself as cancer. I ask myself, what is it here to teach me?

What is your chronic condition teaching you? When you answer that question, and it can take a while, your life begins to truly shift in the direction of choosing to live your life like the gift that it is. ▪

Self-care starts with loving yourself— every part of you.

You must process what is happening to you. It is essential to your healing. It is a beautiful lesson. When you give yourself the time and the space to truly *be* with yourself in full acceptance of where you are, love comes in. When you allow yourself to feel vulnerable and understand what your body is telling you, you can begin to love it. You haven't lost your connection to your body; you just need to give extra tender-loving care to that beautiful vessel that is your home so you can get in sync with each other again. Your body is your house in which you live, and you need to love and nurture it accordingly.

Think about being in an ideal mother-child relationship with your compromised body. If you are a mother and your child is sick, you will do what it takes to make your child better. You reassure her that she is safe and you're doing everything possible to help her get better with patience and presence and ease. This is unconditional love. You would never say, "This is a drag. I'm outta here." So think of your ailing body as your child. Love it, nurture it, soothe it, and be patient with

it. Your body needs to relearn what is essential for it to work properly. This requires your time, your attention, and your devotion to both your soul and your physical being.

Your condition isn't something you choose, but it is something you have. And it is something you need to love in order to heal your life.

This doesn't just go for illnesses. You know how it goes in our everyday lives: over and over again we will commit, commit, commit, *commit* to people and appointments and plans. Before we know it, we have not one weeknight to ourselves. Not one. Then we look around like, "Aw, man, how did that happen?" When that happens, we have to take a good look in the mirror. We planned it. We did that to ourselves. We give to this one, give to that one, and then we are flat on the floor, exhausted. When we run ourselves ragged, we invite illness in the front door.

When we are tired and frazzled, we feel like we want to cancel everything. We want to flake; we want to high five when

Your body is your house in which you live, and you need to love and nurture it accordingly.

someone cancels on us. And then we feel guilty because we're not showing up in the way our family and friends need us to. So we are doing this, that, and the other and sucking at it. We suck at life. Who needs or wants that? I know it may sound foreign or selfish, but if we aren't in tiptop shape, how can we be the best friend, the best daughter, the best mother, the best anyone, for other people? If we don't have any fuel for ourselves, we have no energy to give to things outside of ourselves. We cannot give away what we don't have. We have to fill up our own gas tank to fuel ourselves first. When we do have the energy to live fully, the energy flows and creates a ripple effect to every relationship you have and everything you do.

Don't Zone Out—Zone *In*

Winding down from the day by taking a long walk, writing in a journal, sipping a cup of hot tea and reading a great book, giving your feet a five-minute massage, or stretching for fifteen minutes are great acts of self-love and self-care that need to be scheduled into your life. If you are like me, who had none of these things in my life for a very long time, you need to start thinking about the small steps you can take that lead to big-time healthy changes. Giving yourself attention can feel very foreign at first, but it is an absolute must. Small steps are not quick-fix Band-Aids;

when practiced over time, small steps lead to important, long-term lifestyle changes. We talk about many of these changes (such as changes in diet and exercise) in depth in later chapters, but here we're going to work on what's bugging you (and bugging you out) about your life right now so you can start to change it.

It is the constant repetition of daily acts of self-care that sets you up for optimal shape—mentally, emotionally, and physically.

Self-care isn't a one-time deal. It's not like you can get strep throat, get one acupuncture treatment, and be cured forever. It is the constant repetition of daily acts of self-care that sets you up for optimal shape—mentally, emotionally, and physically. With your focus on self-care, and the repetition of it, the fog will clear, and you will have a new, clear view of the world and everything in it.

Knowing what kinds of things make you feel good makes it easier to immediately start adding them into your week. Self-care looks different for everyone. My partner feels most at peace when he's strumming his guitar or teaching himself how to play a song on the piano. For me, self-care can be as simple as calling up my bestie from college and cracking up with her over something silly. Other people find disconnecting from their cell phone and taking a long walk is helpful. Sometimes (guilty) I like to binge-watch a TV show on Netflix or watch Super Soul Sunday for hours. I also sometimes take FaceTime dance breaks with a friend; we set up our phones so we can see each other, blast a song we love, and dance. Then we hang up and go back to our days.

These are very simple things. I want you to understand that self-care does not need to be overwhelming. You are simply taking the time to mindfully do something that makes you feel great, something that's just for you.

"I breathe music and love to sing as loud and as often as I can (mostly in the car). Music is my go-to, no matter what emotion I'm experiencing. It's my answer to celebration, sadness, connection, and grounding. I constantly need to have music playing, and I need to sing to it always."

Paige Marmer

Sitting in stillness for ninety seconds, deep breathing, or getting in a yogic child's pose for a moment are practices that can have long-lasting value when done intentionally, and doing them regularly can easily turn them into habits.

Commit to scheduling at least one act of self-care a day for three weeks and see what happens. Have a check-in with your bod and your soul, and ask, "How we doing now?" Your body is constantly giving you feedback, advice, and guidance. It is always giving you tips for how to take care of it and what it needs from you. The key is slowing down and tuning in. When you give yourself the space to just be, you give yourself that tune-in time.

Feel-Better Body Scan

Doing a body scan is like taking a deeply relaxing, restorative mini-vacation—right at home, for free, anytime you want! It gives you a chance to identify and release any tension you feel in your body, so that you can stress *less*. The focus required for a body scan keeps your mind from wandering to stressful thoughts, while at the same time brings your attention to the parts of your body that are holding tension.

To begin, put on some pleasant but non-distracting music or sounds of the ocean. Sit or lie down in a very relaxed but supported position and do the simple meditative breathing described on page 22. This helps you get centered and comfortable. I also recommend picturing yourself on a tropical beach, with foamy waves gently enveloping your feet, your thighs, and so on. Feel the warmth—luxuriate in it. Imagine you are bathed in a warm golden light.

Now begin a full body scan. Start by addressing the top, or crown, of your head. Do you notice any tension or tightness? If so, keep your attention there for a moment, and note what you are feeling. Focus on any uncomfortable sensations, and breathe into them using the simple breathing meditation technique. You may feel the tension or pain become more intense and then slowly dissipate.

Repeat this step for your neck; your shoulders; your right arm, hand, and fingers; your upper chest; and your left arm, hand, and fingers. Move down to your abdomen, then your hips, then your right thigh, knee, calf, foot and toes, and then your left thigh, knee, calf, foot, and toes. All along the way, notice any tightness, pain, or pressure. Breathe through the feelings, without judgment, and notice what happens.

If and when other thoughts start vying for attention (and they inevitably will), be polite and acknowledge them, but then send them on their way: *I have to pick up my dry-cleaning before Saturday! Oh, that's interesting. See ya! I wonder what my boss is going to say to me*

on Monday about that report I wrote. We can wonder about that later. Bye-bye. Just acknowledge the thoughts, visualizing them floating away in front of you, and get back to being present in your body scan.

When you have completed the full body scan, you should be deeply relaxed but not asleep. (Well, you might fall asleep, and that's okay too.) Stay there, with your mind clear.

When you are ready to end your session, slowly move or wiggle your toes and gently move your feet back and forth. If you are lying down, bring your knees up to your chest, move each shoulder up and down, and gently shake your hands out. Turn your head from side to side, gently stretching your neck. Open your eyes. Put your hand on your heart and feel it beating. Breathe deeply for a few seconds before standing up and moving into your next activity.

> "Self-care means meditation and mindful breathing exercises for me, even if it's just two minutes a day. It sounds simplistic, but it's not. Don't underestimate the small things. Taking a two- to five-minute session to sit in peace and breathe helps me realize I am safe and well."
>
> *Jennifer Fugo*

Tapping Magic

Emotional Freedom Technique, or EFT, otherwise known as tapping, is a very cool and effective technique to add to your self-care toolbox. Also known as meridian tapping, it involves tapping on specific meridian points on your upper body with your fingertips. Meridian points are part of traditional Chinese medicine. Our life energy, known as *Qi* (pronounced "chee"), flows through our meridians, energetic lines or pathways that run throughout our body. Tapping specific points along these meridians helps release the Qi and, in doing so, relieves stress and anxiety.

Tapping can be learned in a matter of minutes and requires no special equipment; just your fingers and a bit of private space is all you need. You can start using tapping immediately for instant relief from stress and challenges in your life. If you are nervous before a doctor's appointment, tap. When you're feeling less than optimal, tap. You can even tap at the beginning and end of each day to set yourself up for success. Many people I know report immediate relief when tapping during stressful times.

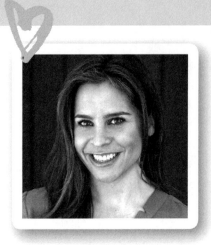

Jessica Ortner

Jessica Ornter is a co-producer of *The Tapping Solution,* a breakthrough documentary film on the Emotional Freedom Technique (EFT), also known as tapping or meridian tapping, and author of the *New York Times* bestselling book *The Tapping Solution for Weight Loss & Body Confidence.*

Here, she shares her thoughts about tapping.

Tapping is a technique in which you use your fingers to tap on meridian points in order to relieve stress. We intuitively know, for example, that the key meridian points near the eyebrows, nose, temple, and chest can comfort us, which is why we often unconsciously touch these areas when we are under stress. Tapping lets us access these points in a conscious and deliberate way.

When we have chronic illness, there are many emotions involved: sadness, frustration over what you are missing out on in life, and so on. For people with physical challenges, the burden of emotions can be paralyzing. You want to get those negative feelings cleared. Tapping is a means of clearing those emotions away and stimulating specific acupressure points, and that in turn sends a calming signal to your brain, telling you that it is safe for you to relax. So you can think about whatever you need to think about without getting hijacked by emotions. Before you plant the seeds of growth, you have to pull the weeds, and tapping supports doing that.

First of all, you need to have clarity on what you want to work on. Maybe today what is bothering you is how you feel when people ask for things you don't have the energy or emotional or physical ability to give. Or it could be that you are upset that you are not getting support you need. *Start where you are:* "I am angry that my friend called and didn't ask how I was doing." "I feel like I have too much on my plate."

If your concern is generic, tapping won't be as effective. Be specific. When it comes to pain, you can begin to tap on the symptom: "Even though my tummy hurts, I love and accept myself." "Even though I have this pain in my lower back, I love and accept myself." The important thing is to give the issue a voice, your voice. Measure on a scale from one to ten how much emotional pain you are in before you start tapping. See if you moved from a ten to a five on the pain meter after doing a tapping sequence. Once you go down to a two or three, you can incorporate other specific statements.

I think it's a good idea to start out using a script. Write down your concern and give yourself five minutes to do one sequence. That's really all it takes. If when you finish you feel you need to do another sequence, repeat it. Or do another one using a different line or script. When you do it as a regular practice, the tapping sequence becomes second nature. ∎

Tapping 101

Before you begin: Choose a very specific emotional focus you would like to clear from your mind. Put that emotional focus into words—for example, "I am angry at myself" or "My diagnosis feels overwhelming."

Now insert that emotional-focus phrase into the following sentence: "Even though I (insert your chosen phrase here), I love and accept myself." For instance:

▶ Even though I am angry that I feel so sick, I love and accept myself.

▶ Even though I'm nervous about seeing this new doctor, I love and accept myself.

▶ Even though I'm mad at myself for not being able to keep up with my friends, I love and accept myself.

▶ Even though I have a rash all over my body, I love and accept myself.

▶ Even though my diagnosis feels overwhelming, I love and accept myself.

Good Morning Rituals

Self-care in the a.m. is essential if you want to set a positive tone for the rest of your day. If you have a bad morning, it's pretty hard to reset the rest of the day to positive. I am a firm believer that a good morning means a great day. When I do not do my morning self-care, I tend to be a little monster. This little monster has been lovingly called "Cramy," a combination of *crazy* and *Amy*. She's my alter ego and not someone I want around. My daily acts of self-care make a huge positive difference in my day: I am more patient, grounded, thoughtful, and present, and I am much more likely to think about decisions and choices.

Here are some morning self-care suggestions:

▶ Start the night before and put your phone on airplane mode before you tuck yourself in. Who wants to wake up to a buzzing, vibrating mobile device filled with texts from the night before?

▶ After rising, do a few gentle stretches to awaken your beautiful bod. You can massage your arms, legs, feet, and hands to wake everything up gently.

▶ Get in the bathroom to do your thing, which for me includes washing my face and brushing my teeth, natch.

▶ Try for twenty minutes of meditation, but if you can only do five to ten minutes, that's okay too. Even ninety seconds is *great* and has a positive effect.

▶ Ease into your day with a cup of hot water and lemon or a calming tea. Take it slow.

The Tapping Sequence

Using two or three fingertips, you will tap on each of the following meridian points, in order, gently and quickly from six to ten times. As you tap, say your full emotional-focus sentence out loud.

POINT 1   The soft side of the hand between the wrist and little finger. Use a karate-chop motion to tap this point.

POINT 2   The point where the inner eyebrow begins.

POINT 3   The outside of the eye, but not touching the eye.

POINT 4   The lower rim of your eye socket directly under your eye.

POINT 5   The fleshy indented area between your nose and upper lip.

POINT 6   The indention on your chin that sits just below your lower lip.

POINT 7   The area about an inch below the lowest edge of your collar or breastbone.

POINT 8   Three to four inches directly under your arm pit, where there is a soft and slightly tender spot.

POINT 9   The crown of your head.

FINISH   After you have completed tapping all nine points, take a moment to reevaluate your emotional state. If you are still intensely or moderately stressed or upset, repeat the sequence two to four more times until your emotions are in control and you are at peace.

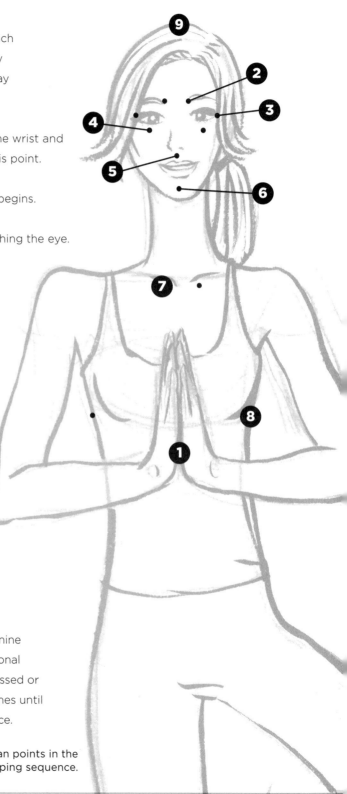

Tap each of these nine meridian points in the numbered order during a tapping sequence.

- Do some very brief journaling. I don't mean create a to-do list and stress bomb yourself. Write out how you are feeling and get any negative emotions or worries out on the paper. Then freewrite your intentions for the day, which can be very simple. For example, I might say, "Today I will carry myself with ease, I will remain calm in any stressful situations, and I will have fun."

- Give yourself a reassuring mirror moment (see page 32).

- Say what you are grateful for. Take note of what you are grateful for in that moment. You can write this down or just think it to yourself. By cultivating an attitude of gratitude, we immediately shift our day into a more positive and happy energy. You'll find that when you take a few minutes to be consciously aware of what makes you grateful—the food on your plate, the roof over your head, the people you love—you shift into a more balanced and awake state, one in which you celebrate your present moment, getting out of your head and into your heart.

Your morning ritual can include any and all of the above. Or you might want to take a morning walk or watch the sun rise if you are an early bird. Maybe a bit of inspirational reading would set you on the right path for the day. Find one or two things you like to do, whatever they are, to set yourself up for a great day and then do them.

Pleasant Evening Rituals

When winding down at the end of the day, add in a few self-care rituals to honor all that you did during the day and to prepare yourself for a well-deserved evening's rest.

- When finishing up your work tasks for the day, write out a to-do list of things you didn't get done and that need to be done tomorrow. Then when you're done with your workday, you are less likely to continue thinking about work.

- Before you enter your home (a.k.a. your Zen den), mindfully say to yourself, "I am choosing to leave behind any stress I picked up during the day today right here and not continue on with it."

- Wipe away any bad energy or stress with a hot shower. If you have time, take a salt bath with an essential oil added. (See pages 46 and 48 for my list of favorite essential oils for baths.)

- About sixty to ninety minutes before bed, turn off *all* electronics, including mobile phones, TVs, tablets, laptops, and other devices.

- Dim the lights (dimmer switches are one of the greatest inventions ever). Light a candle. Put on some soft, restful music. Slow it on down.

- Repeat some gentle stretches from the morning.

- Read something uplifting or journal about something positive.

- Take note of what you were grateful for in the day to help yourself wind down in a peaceful way.

Be an Earth Mama

Anything you can do to ground yourself, or be fully conscious and present in the moment, is an important aspect of self-care. For instance, sit with your spine directly against the wall and practice the simple meditative breathing exercise on page 22. Dance for a minute or two. Lie in savasana (corpse pose, where you lie on your back, arms and legs spread at forty-five degrees). Do some gentle yoga stretches. Smell some grounding essential oils, which produce natural feel-good serotonin. Do a squat against the wall; place your hand on your belly, and do deep breathing. Feel your breath as it drops low into your belly.

Connecting to the earth helps. Take a fifteen-minute walk to get some much-needed sunshine and soak in some Vitamin D. Sit under a tree and watch the leaves dance in the wind.

Schedule these mini but *mucho* important grounding activities into your day because it's way too easy to let them slide if you don't. If dancing or yoga helps you feel more grounded and present in your body, hold out ten minutes for them anytime during the day. If walking is what makes you feel connected to the earth and nature, block out fifteen minutes on your calendar for it.

Whatever you choose to do, do it with the intention to help yourself be present and to see yourself as an important part of the world or the universe. When you're out for a walk, for example, don't just hustle from point A to point B, like you might when walking to get somewhere. Lift up your head and notice what's around you. Take in the sky, the people near you, the trees as they move in the wind. Feel the breeze on your face; notice the beautiful colors of the seasonal leaves all over the ground. Be present in your surroundings and take a couple long deep breaths. Take a time out to tune in to nature or your environment.

Baby Your Bod

Being good to the curvy container that holds your heart and soul, not to mention all the miraculous workings of your amazing body, is right up there with showing respect for your elders and kindness toward children and animals. It's not something you want to play around with. How could you not respect the incredible organism, your body, that knows to sweat to cool you off when it's hot and that can heal itself when you get a scrape? The good news is the body is so wonderfully enjoyable to take care of. Especially for those of us who contend with the stress of chronic illness, making nice with the body that works so hard for us is the least we can do. There are many body-care rituals I could talk about, but here are a few of my favorites.

Aromatherapy

We've all experienced the power of scent and how it can shift our mood and energy in the matter of a sniff. You know how B.O. makes you quietly but quickly move away from the stinky guy on your morning train? Or how the smell of cookies baking makes you feel all warm and happy inside? Then you understand the power of scent.

Aromatherapy is the targeted use of aromatic, natural plant oils and extracts to lift your mood and increase your cognitive, psychological, and physical well-being. Scientists and researchers believe that odor detection receptors in our nose communicate with parts of our brain, specifically the parts that hold memories and emotions. Smelling essential oils can make you feel instantly relaxed and centered.

Be sure to use pure, organic essential oils. Synthetic oils don't have the same natural and pleasant aroma or the healing powers of the real thing. Many scented products on the market advertised as "therapeutic" actually contain synthetic products. They're fakers! Read labels carefully. Who likes a phony?

One of my favorite things to do is put relaxing oil on my wrists or my temples and breathe it in. Just be sure to read the label on your oil before applying it to your skin; some need to be mixed with neutral or carrier oil before touching your skin.

Here are some of my favorite oils and oil blends:

▸ To feel more balanced when you're stressed, you can try lavender, ylang-ylang, frankincense, spruce, ho wood, or chamomile.

▸ To soothe sore muscles and joints, give these a try: wintergreen, camphor, peppermint, blue tansy, chamomile, helichrysum.

▸ For respiratory health, try eucalyptus oil. It also helps relieve sore muscles when added to the bath.

- When you need a pick-me-up or a mood boost, any citrus essential oil, like orange or grapefruit, is a great idea. They are energizing and revitalizing. Peppermint is also a great pick-me-up. (Plus, it is great for digestion.) All are good choices when you're feeling like a couch potato.

- Lavender essential oil is a great way to help you wind down from the day or relax at a moment's notice. It's like Xanax, but not dangerously habit forming. Its relaxing and anti-anxiety properties help you sleep better.[2] You can put a drop on your pillow before bed. Happy snoozing!

Brush-Up Your Skin

Our skin is our body's largest organ! It performs many functions that are crucial for our health: It shields us from germs and sends signals to our body's immune system to spring into action when germs have attacked. It helps regulate body temperature. Nerve endings in the skin send signals to our brain about what we are feeling when we pet a dog, touch a hot kettle, or stick our bare hand in snow.

For all the things skin does for us, we should do something for it, aside from applying chemical-filled moisturizer and sunscreen. Dry brushing is simple and quick way to keep your skin in great shape and for waking up your tired body. It is detoxifying, which people who have chronic health issues often need

extra help with. Brushing with a natural-bristle brush exfoliates dry, flaky skin, and stimulates both blood circulation and your lymphatic system. It also helps with cellulite (woot woot!).

You will need a new, clean natural-bristle brush. Get one with a long detachable handle, so you can reach all areas of your body. These brushes are generally found in the bath and body section of good health food stores. Here's what you do with it:

1 Before you bathe or shower, remove your clothing and stand on a bathmat or in the shower. Detach the brush handle, so you're holding just the bristle part in your hand.

2 Very gently brush your skin, starting at your feet. Move the brush in long, circular motions up your ankle, calves, and thighs, making sure to always move up and toward your heart. Never brush in a downward movement.

3 Overlap brushing areas as you move, working on one leg and then the other, one arm and then the other, and then your torso. Don't dry brush your face and be gentle around sensitive areas.

4 Reattach the handle of the brush. Now brush your back in an upward motion.

5 When you are done, rinse off in a hot shower. Doing a final rinse in cool water will further stimulate blood circulation. *Voila!*

"Self-care is a huge part of my health and overall wellness. I'm a very routine-oriented person, and I like to stick to things when they make me feel good. I like to start and end my day the same way, like bookends. I've got a fifteen-minute routine where I start off with a silent meditation in my bed, thinking about the day ahead and organizing my thoughts. Afterward, I cleanse my face, brush my teeth, use mouthwash, apply moisturizer and eye cream, and floss. Mentally and physically, I feel renewed, centered, and grounded through this process. My nighttime routine is the same, except I end with the silent meditation in bed. No day starts or ends without this!"

Tara Sowlaty

Bathing Beauty

I absolutely love a hot bath. My friend recently said that he could create a really good drinking game (with green juice, of course) for every time I say "Epsom salts." What's not to like? A hot bath with Epsom salts helps your muscles relax and can help ease headaches, cramps, backaches, and knots in shoulder and neck muscles. It also gets you sweating, which is detoxifying for your body. The psychological benefits of a relaxing soak can't be underestimated, either.

Here's my favorite Epsom salt bath recipe. Fill your tub with comfortably warm water. (Super hot water can dry out your skin and strip away protective oils.) Pour in two heaping cups of Epsom salt. Add in four to five drops of lavender essential oil (or any other relaxing scent you like), and soak for twenty to forty minutes. This bath is extremely detoxifying; it helps you work up a sweat, and this allows enough time for your body to remove the toxins and to absorb the salt's minerals, magnesium, and sulfate. You feel deliciously at peace when you're done.

Here are some other tips for getting the most from your bath time:

▸ Keep it quiet, relaxing, and uninterrupted. That means turn off your phone and TV. Put on some soothing music (no talk radio!).

▸ Light candles, dim the lights, and wind the room down so you can wind down.

▸ Adding essential oils to your bath boosts the power of the tub. To de-stress at the end of the day or on a leisurely weekend, add two to three drops of an essential oil (lavender is the most relaxing) to the warm running water as you fill the tub.

▸ When you're in the tub, lie back and let your mind wander—or just let go of all the worries of the day.

▸ An unhurried hot bath can raise your temperature slightly. When you leave the tub, the rapid cool off your body experiences tells your brain it's sleepy time.[3]

Slumber Party

According to the National Sleep Foundation, adult women (from twenty-six to sixty-four years old) should get a minimum of seven to nine hours of sleep per night.[4] For too many women, however—and I used to be one of them—the idea of a good night's sleep is pretty alien. We wake up feeling tired and never feel fully rested after a night in bed. It's such a disservice to our health and well-being to deprive our bodies and brains of a deep, restorative sleep.

Electronic devices, external lights and noise from the street, televisions, radios, alarm clocks, and other sources interfere with our circadian rhythm or our natural sleep-wake cycle. Even if we don't notice these things, or tell ourselves we don't, our body knows about them and fights back while we're trying to sleep. That's when we feel exhausted and draggy during the day. Don't make bad sleep another chronic issue to deal with.

Here's how to get a good night's sleep:

DE-CLUTTER YOUR BEDROOM. Make it your sanctuary. Get rid of anything that makes you stressed out or that impedes your movement into and out of bed. Less is more in the bedroom. Choose a soothing color for the wall.

MAKE YOUR BED COMFY. A good mattress that suits your body but offers back and neck support is the first step in making your bed a beautiful place to be. Soft, clean sheets and a big, cozy comforter are also fundamental. Big, soft pillows offer good head and neck support and help you breathe easy. You want to feel like you are hopping into a cloud.

"My bedroom is set up for a good night's rest. One of my top priorities is to make my bed the most comfortable place possible. I am very affected by environment, so keeping my house neat is important. I make sure I have my own space: my bedroom that is clean and really nice. I have really good, soft sheets and beautiful blankets and pillows. It's nice to know you can crawl into a cloud-like, comforting nest at the end of a rough day—or any day."

Kaitlyn Lennon

STICK TO A REGULAR BEDTIME.
Remember when Mom tucked you in at
8:00 p.m. on school nights? She was a pretty
smart cookie. Getting to bed at the same
time each night is a healthy routine that
will eventually get your mind and body into
sync when it's time to hit the sack. Choose
a time when you generally start to feel tired.
Pushing yourself past that period can actually
hurt your chances of falling asleep quickly.
For me, it's 10:00 p.m. and lights out. Some
people need to go to bed earlier; for others,
11:00 p.m. works. Remember to build in at
least half an hour for your unrushed evening
self-care routine.

WAKE UP AT THE SAME TIME EVERY DAY.
If you're going to bed at the same time
every night, and falling asleep and staying
asleep, then you should wake up naturally
at the same time every morning without the
help of your cell phone or alarm clock. If
you need a nudge in the beginning, set your
alarm to play some soothing tunes, *not* a
fire-alarm sound.

DON'T EAT TOO LATE. Eat at least three
hours before you plan to go to bed. So for
example, if lights out are at 10:00 p.m.,
dinner should be no later than 7:00 p.m.

LISTEN TO YOUR BODY. Your body knows
what's up. If you're tired, go to bed! Don't
resist and then end up on the insomnia train
to nowhere.

DON'T GO TO BED MAD. If you want to
set yourself up for a fun night of no sleep,
then be sure to keep every emotion, feeling,
and experience from the day all pent up
inside. However, if you want to have a
blissful slumber, you should let it all out in
a peaceful and effective way. If something
really bugged you during the day, write the
problem out in your journal. Unloading
problems onto a piece of paper will move
them out of your head, which is crucial if
you want to get some Z's. Don't wait until
bedtime to get something off your chest.
Otherwise you'll be tossing and turning
your pretty head all night.

GROOVE TO A SOUND MACHINE.
A sound or white-noise machine helps
neutralize environmental sounds that
might bother you, from your partner's
snoring to traffic noise on the street to a
heating system that clangs all night. The
sound these small boxes produce is a gentle
wooshing that cancels out everything else
and helps you sleep more soundly.

Getting into the Self-Care Habit

My self-care routine is deceptively simple and effective because it pays me back one hundredfold in a sense of well-being and centeredness. To help yourself get into a new self-care-minded lifestyle routine, schedule in ways to remind yourself of what your end goal is: to take better care of you. Giving yourself gentle reminders throughout the day is a good place to start. Try setting a reminder alert to ring on your phone several times throughout the day that says, "What have I done to take care of myself today?" Or place sticky notes around your house with loving affirmations that gently nudge you in the way of taking action for you. You can literally write "Love yourself" or "What are you doing for you?" and put them all over your house so you can start to slow down and incorporate them. Visually seeing these reminders will help you stop, drop, and breathe and have a much needed check-in with yourself.

Use your daily reminders and take note of your new healthy choices—and then give yourself a pat on the back for taking care of yourself. You'll soon find it's extremely satisfying and rewarding to take care of you.

4

Be Your Own Best Advocate

I went to the School of Hard Knocks when it came to learning how to find, choose, and work with the right doctors and other health care practitioners. You're looking at someone who went to thirty (ten as a child and twenty-five as a young adult) doctors before she was thirty. Nope, I'm not kidding. I've tried *everything* and crossed the health care map many times between holistic and conventional medicine. Did my health care providers always have my best interests in mind? Sometimes. But they all handed me big bills before saying, "Bye, have a nice day!" That's the unfortunate truth about much of today's health care landscape: you pull out your checkbook no matter what kind of care you did (or didn't) receive.

Still, it's important to find the right doctors, even if it means making appointments and giving them a test run. While that sounds daunting (and potentially expensive), it's worse and more costly, in so many ways, to stay with a doctor or practitioner who misdiagnoses your issue or doesn't understand it and, as a result, can't launch you on your journey to health.

Becoming your own best healer goes beyond the self-care we dished about in the previous chapter. You know your body better than anyone. You must become an educated health consumer. Find out as much as you can about your condition. Don't be intimidated, and don't stop asking thoughtful questions. You have to put yourself first, even on bad days. You are not a helpless victim. *You* are in control of your own destiny.

What I Learned from the Wrong Docs

When I moved back home after my trip to Israel, the first doctor I saw was my childhood general practitioner. I hadn't seen her in years. The first thing she did was a blood workup. I thought I had some terminal illness (of course!). Anxiety (check!) and worry (check!) helped me create all sorts of devastating scenarios: I have cancer. I'm dying. I'm going to have to get a whole body transplant. When the blood-test results came back, I asked her what was wrong with me. Her answer didn't come as a relief. "Well, everything," she said. I know now that this is a response people with chronic conditions hear quite often. It's not helpful, to say the least.

My next stop on the fast-moving health care conveyer belt was a highly recommended gastroenterologist (GI doc) at a prominent hospital. I was so swollen I could barely open my mouth to smile, I had hives and rashes all over my body, my hair was falling out in clumps, I wasn't absorbing nutrients, and I had deep pain in my intestines. I couldn't even stand straight, I couldn't keep anything but liquids down, I was almost in need of a wheelchair I was so weak, and above all else I hadn't gone to the bathroom in one full month. Yet this doctor basically told me I was fine, that food allergies don't matter, and that I should take a medication for bad gut bacteria for a couple days and see her again in ten to twelve weeks. Say what? Yup, that's what happened. And she was supposed to the best in the biz. There is no other way to feel but depressed and hopeless in a moment like that.

In my desperation, which was getting worse by the day, I went to see another doctor, a family practitioner with a newfound interest in holistic medicine. He was a good salesman. Let's call him Dr. Cure-All. At the time he sounded exactly like the kind of doctor I needed. I liked him; he was nice and caring, and it seemed to me at the time—mind you, this is when I had no knowledge of the health

care game—that he could just handle everything. Why? *Because he told me he could.* I'd grown up believing a good doctor would just find the right pill and make you all better. Besides, with all of my past experience with pill popping to solve problems, a doctor who talked about herbs and the whole body working as a system sounded much more appealing.

I trusted him. I was overwhelmed and frightened, my body was in a state of emergency, and no one I had seen so far had a handle on what was happening to me. I was so weak and so sick, with not a spark of energy left. And to be brutally honest, I wanted someone else to just handle it for me. This was before I understood that no one would or could handle *me* better than myself. I wanted someone to guide me, not understanding then that that someone was *Amy.* I felt like a speeding train that was running out of steam, slowing down, chugging sideways as it ran out of gas, and finally drifting off the tracks toward the cliff. I was desperate, and I put my trust in him. I wish I could reach back to my naïve, terrified, and deeply pained twenty-five-year-old self and give her a hug, sweetly and softly, and say, "Amy. You got this. You can connect with yourself and *know* what is right. You know what *feels* right."

Dr. Cure-All treated me with thyroid medication because my thyroid was struggling after my trip abroad. The medication made me feel so much better, as it would anyone with an underactive thyroid. But it was never enough because there were underlying problems that weren't being addressed. Dr. Cure-All, it turned out, didn't walk his talk. Instead, of looking at my body as a whole, he kept raising my dose of thyroid medicine. And I was raising my ability to do things I hadn't been able to do, not realizing that he was making a perfect storm into a hurricane. It wasn't until a full year of my thyroid meds getting higher and higher that I realized something was *seriously* wrong with me.

The eye of the storm had passed over me, and I felt as though I had been swept into the cyclone. One morning I woke up feeling as though I was having a full-blown panic attack. My body was in *Amy-you-have-to-handle-this* mode. I somehow got my ass in a cab and made it to the office of my local internist, unable to breathe, panting for air, dripping in sweat, eyes blurry and bugging out of my head. They immediately took my vitals and hooked me up to an oxygen tank.

Starting Over

I knew something had to change, starting with Dr. Cure-All. I had heard a well-known doctor of functional medicine speak several years back when I was seemingly healthy. He was impressive and made a lasting impression. I had wanted to see him years before

You know your body better than anyone.

Dr. Cure-All had come into the picture, but I hadn't listened to my second brain (a.k.a. my gut) when it nudged me in that direction. Now I used any and every connection I had to reach out to him. After all, what did I have to lose? Oh right, *my life*.

He agreed to take my case on. My mom, boyfriend, and I packed our bags and trekked up north to his office in Massachusetts.

With the sweetest and gentlest smile, he hugged me hello, and my mom, boyfriend, and I all instinctively and simultaneously breathed a huge deep sigh of relief. In that moment, the three of us each felt that we were in the right place. I was so thankful that I'd finally listened to my inner guide.

It was the first time I didn't feel like I was just another patient in another cold, sterile medical office. This doctor *saw* me. He ran tests I had never even heard of. He immediately set me up with nutritional IVs and shots to help boost my ability to absorb the minerals and vitamins I was depleted in. I started to feel better. I still had a very, very long road ahead of me, but I knew in my gut that I was supposed to be on this journey with this doctor and that I was finally heading in the right direction. I knew that I was finally *safe*. He showed me that I can't just be diagnosed with everything; every part of the body works together, and if nothing is working, something needed to be the root cause.

This doctor was the first one to look at my case and all of my health issues in a holistic, or systemic, way. As a functional medicine practitioner, he was the first one who looked at *all* of my symptoms and put them together like an intricate puzzle. His knowledge and the way he explained my case were so impressive. He simultaneously prescribed conventional pharmaceutical medication, as needed, and focused on lifestyle and natural ways of healing. He offered a new way of thinking and understanding my health, but I was aware that my inner guide had been trying to tell me something similar. Popping a pill or just taking herbs wasn't going to cut it in my situation; it never cut it in the first place. Those of us in the Chronic Condition

Seek out doctors who see you as an individual, rather than a case file, and see your condition as something to truly manage and heal, rather than as a diagnosis to medicate.

Club, or CC Club, need someone who looks at our entire system, pulls information from both Eastern and Western philosophies and treatments, and puts a strong emphasis on lifestyle and diet. My intuition had been trying to tell me this for a long time, but I hadn't been listening.

The reason I felt I always needed more medicine was because Dr. Cure-All wasn't dealing with my underlying parasite, celiac, malnutrition, colon issues, and heavy metal issues. With the help of my new functional medicine doctor and my thyroid specialist, I learned that I was being overmedicated with thyroid-stimulating hormones—dangerously so. Dr. Cure-All had literally given me artificial Graves disease, an autoimmune disease that affects the thyroid, and I was lucky my heart hadn't stopped. (A normal heart rate is 60 to 80 resting, and with the "help" I'd received from Dr. Cure-All, mine was 110 resting.)

As my two new doctors began to taper off the thyroid meds Dr. Cure-All had me on, my body went through withdrawal and had a tough time adjusting. The word *scary* doesn't even cover it. Every single day I had to use an oxygen tank. I was sweating and then freezing. I was panting for air, and I was shaky. My hormones were raging (literally—I was acting like an alpha male hopped up on too much testosterone, willing to fight with anyone who looked at me the wrong way). I was exhausted and depleted one minute and revved up and speeding the very next. My heart felt like it was going to burst out of my chest. To this day, I'm still not taking a normal dose of thyroid meds, and I need a check-up every month to make sure I am stable.

So what did I learn from this experience? By not taking charge of my own condition, not taking care of myself, and not listening to my original gut instinct that told me to seek out another doctor, I had wasted a lot of precious time and put myself at serious, life-altering risk.

When I was seeing Dr. Cure-All, I was so wrapped up in my dramatic symptoms that I was not asking questions, and the biggest question I wasn't asking myself was, "Do you like this doctor simply because he is telling you what you want to hear?" I put all of my faith into someone because he was nice to me and told me he knew what to do. His treatment was masking my condition just like the pain pills did when I was a kid. This was a life-threatening lesson that majorly set my healing back. I felt sad about the fact that I hadn't taken better care of myself, and it was in this moment that I realized my mistake and I started to learn how to do that. I also learned early on that if I didn't do the work to get to the right people, I could live in a scary place for a very long time and feel like a powerless victim.

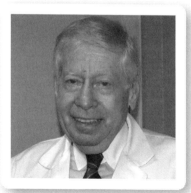

Philip Felig, MD

Philip Felig, MD, is an endocrinologist in New York City. His expertise has been recognized in *New York Magazine's* "Best Doctors" list thirteen times. He has also been designated as an outstanding endocrinologist by the Consumer's Research Council of America. He attended the Yale University School of Medicine and was awarded the Anatomy Prize and the Campbell Prize for highest standing in the exams.

Thyroid issues are incredibly common, especially in women, and many of us in the Chronic Condition Club have thyroid issues in addition to other ▸

conditions. Because thyroid issues are so prevalent and require precise care (as I learned the hard way), I asked Dr. Felig, the endocrinologist on my A-team, to give us a little bit of thyroiducation. Knowing how your thyroid works, how its function is tested, and how thyroid issues can be treated is essential knowledge if you're to be the best advocate for your thyroid health. Hypothyroidism was a major player for me. Here are some ways you can see if it could be part of your condition as well.

The primary function of the thyroid gland is to regulate the metabolism. The thyroid makes two hormones. If there are not enough thyroid hormones, the metabolism is likely to be slowed down, and people may feel tired or fatigued. This can affect their mood; they can feel depressed, and they may also gain weight. On the other side of the coin, if the thyroid is overactive, people feel sped up, and they may feel anxious. They are often aware of their heart pounding or shakiness. If somebody is having symptoms such as fatigue or weakness, weight gain, decreased appetite, change in menstrual periods, loss of sex drive, feeling cold when others don't, or constipation, and there is no other logical explanation, they should have their thyroid checked as a possible factor in these symptoms.

The immune system is often to blame when the thyroid malfunctions. This is the part of the body that protects us against foreign invaders. But some people have antibodies that stimulate the thyroid; this can lead to an overactive thyroid. More commonly, however, the antibodies may interfere with the thyroid, resulting in an underactive thyroid.

It is crucial for good health to have your thyroid in balance. But you might not be aware of the symptoms of thyroid imbalance or might attribute these symptoms to other conditions. So while not everyone needs to have their entire endocrine system checked, most people who have an annual exam should get a thyroid-screening test to measure the TSH, or thyroid-stimulating hormone. If the TSH is elevated, pointing to an underactive thyroid, measuring the two hormones, T4 or Free T4 and the T3 or the Free T3, gives us additional information useful in delivering treatment. Thyroid issues can often be ruled out if the TSH is within normal limits.

If you do have an issue with your thyroid, it's crucial to work closely with a doctor or a specialist with expertise in the area of endocrinology. Otherwise you could be at risk for inadequate and inappropriate treatment, as well as an imbalance in your overall health. ■

Finding *Your* Perfect Doctor(s)

Those of us who have chronic health conditions likely don't fit into a standard doctor's patient blueprint or have an easily identifiable problem that has a prescribed treatment (that the doc learned about in medical school). Few doctors are trained to automatically look for and understand chronic conditions and how to get to the root of what is causing our symptoms. *Your* symptoms can sound like a dozen different issues to someone who doesn't have the training in or experience with people who have multiple health issues. Two must-have qualifications your doctor should possess are the ability to diagnose your issue correctly *and* the ability to create the right plan of action for your care, including providing medicine, supplements, diet and lifestyle recommendations, and physical and emotional therapy options tailored to your individual needs.

Ideally, we need to seek guidance from people who are ready and available (and excited) to look outside the standard patient's ailments to find out what the root cause of our condition is. This is just one more reason to seek out doctors who see you as an individual, rather than a case file, and see your condition as something to truly manage and heal, rather than as a diagnosis to medicate.

A personal connection with your doctor is so important when you have chronic health challenges. When you are on the chronic-conditions spectrum, it is easy for practitioners to make you feel like you must be doing something to make yourself unwell, that maybe it's all in your head, or you were directly harming yourself. (Huh? Say what?) It is also often hard to find a doctor who has time to look up from your case file to look *you* in the eye for more than ten seconds, take you in, and really connect on a human level. I have met people who have actually stopped looking for doctors because they've become so discouraged about the callous "Next!" attitude of the health care system. They practice the best self-care they can muster under these circumstances, but they shouldn't have to do that. Neither should you.

> *Not only can doctors be wrong, but also they can simply be wrong for you.*

There is a power that doctors have, what with their white lab coats, charts, and stethoscopes. It's as if that white coat gives them some magic ability to answer every question correctly and decide your fate with the swipe of a tongue depressor. But no doctor has magical powers. Not only can doctors be wrong, but also they can simply be wrong *for you. And that's okay.*

Finding a doctor is like making any important decision in life. Do you hire the first person who walks into a job interview? Would you buy or rent the first apartment you see? Of course not. You want to work with people who give you the right quality of work and attention, and you want to live in a place that makes you feel safe and at ease. Feel free to hire and fire when necessary.

Finally, regular gut checks are important because the gut is your second brain, and it is often much more direct than what your brain is telling you. If one doctor just doesn't feel like the right fit for you, or if your gut is telling you another doc might be, heed that message.

> "In the beginning, soon after I was diagnosed with Crohn's disease, I saw a doctor who didn't totally get it. So I was on the wrong meds for a while, and my liver was crazy. It just was not working out, so we asked for referrals from other doctors, and we got to the right place because of it."
>
> *Tara Sowlaty*

Start by Ruling Things Out

When you have a complicated health situation and you aren't sure what the hell is going on, the most powerful place you can start from is ruling things out. I can tell you this with certainty because after my bucket load of bad doctor experiences, I went to all sorts of health care providers, including all sorts of specialists, to make sure I didn't have a condition that was actively destructive to my body. I put on my detective badge and made sure I wasn't missing anything.

You are the boss. No one cares more about your healing than you.

I broke out in hives, and my immune markers were high, so I went to an immunologist. Things came back normal because it wasn't my immune system that was causing those symptoms. *Check.*

I had symptoms that indicated a parasite issue, so I went to a parasitologist. He found not one but two infections. Oh, I have a worm infection, you say? *Whip worm and its entire family?* And it's bad? That could explain why my hair is falling out, why I feel so weak, why I'm itching everywhere, why I'm dropping weight for no reason, and why I'm having all sorts of uncomfortable bowel issues? Exterminator needed! Knock those fuckers out! *Check.* Treated it.

Every time I did a "check," and even if it revealed something, as the parasitologist did, I felt better. I could understand what was happening. I was in control.

I dare you to try it! The more you rule things out, the less stress you will have. When it comes to illness, the big black hole of the unknown is frightening and debilitating. The more you can rule out, the better you will feel and therefore the more in control you will be.

Set the Ground Rules

Don't get it twisted: You are the captain of your ship. No one cares more about your healing than you. You don't have to settle for the get-'em-in-and-get-'em-out attitude that some physicians with crowded waiting rooms and too much paperwork (often through no fault of their own) offer. You have every right to let doctors know your concerns and experiences, good and bad. Otherwise, they can't help you during subsequent appointments, and you may carry a festering grudge. You also need to make sure you and the doctor are a good match because the end goal is partnering well with your doctor on your quest for healing. Think "team"!

I had gotten most of my issues under control until my colon was the only thing

> "You can't be superwoman. Needing and forming a good support system doesn't mean we are victims. It means we are human."
>
> *Lindsay White*

left in the equation that didn't seem to be working properly. After the first specialist at my rock-bottom moment told me I would have to have my colon removed, I went to see a very well-established colorectal surgeon for a second opinion. He came very highly recommended from many people I trust and respect. Since he was highly specialized, my insurance did not cover the visit, so I paid out of pocket. He was the best, and when you are in the territory of complexity that my condition presented, more often than not, you have to go to specialists who don't take insurance, or at least not your insurance. My first visit would cost $1,000 *if* it didn't include any tests.

I liked the doctor immediately; I felt he was very present. When I went to the clinic that did the specific test he had prescribed, a test to find out why I wasn't eliminating properly, I was quite nervous. What I didn't realize was just how traumatizing a pelvic-floor examination can be when not done with care. The procedure is by nature invasive and embarrassing. Moreover, it is most often done on older women. The youngish doctor doing my test was unnerved when he met me. It was immediately apparent that he was clearly not expecting someone in her early thirties. This made him uncomfortable, and that in turn made me feel very unsafe and vulnerable. It would have been a real plus to have had a doctor who had some experience dealing with patients younger than eighty.

When I tried to get back in touch with the doctor who prescribed the test to let him know what had happened, his office took a message and said he'd call me back. But he never did. Doctors often don't know what their front office is doing with phone calls from patients. They trust the nurses and administrative assistants at the reception desk to deal with patients, but they are not always aware of how that's being done. I actually had to schedule another follow-up appointment—and pay $500 for that—just to get in front of him to tell him about the experience. I felt very depressed and horrible about my experience, the difficulty getting in touch with the doctor, and having to pay to tell him what happened, so I dreaded the appointment and had a lot of anxiety about it.

When I talked to my therapist (yup, I'm on the couch too), he and I went over what I should say when I went into the doctor's office for the follow-up appointment. So when I got in to see the colorectal doctor, I was able to tell him clearly, calmly, and very politely about the horrible experience I had had. I described it to him in detail, and I told him I'd tried but failed to get him on the phone to tell him about it.

Then I said, "I'm fighting for my life and have been for five years. If you don't have the time to commit to me as a patient and partner with me, it's totally, 100 percent okay. I need to know either way now so I can find someone else who does have the time if you don't. I truly want to work with you and have you as my doctor. I simply don't have the energy to chase anyone. I have been through so much, and I need to partner with someone who will make my care a priority. And I hope that it can be you."

His head snapped back and spun around on his neck, sort of like Linda Blair in the *Exorcist,* but without the makeup or the pea soup. Then he genuinely apologized and gave me his cell phone number. He has been 100 percent responsive ever since.

I took away two important lessons from this experience. First, by stating what I needed clearly and calmly, I was able to see if, based on his response, he was truly the right doctor for me. Second, I learned that if you don't get on the court, it is easy to stay a victim of your circumstance, especially when it comes to your health care.

Create Your Health Care A-Team

Nothing feels worse than going through a crisis and feeling totally out of control and alone. If you are in the Chronic Condition Club and you willingly go through the same loop of unhelpful crisis-mode behaviors every single time shit hits the fan, it's like you are willingly jumping off a bridge. You don't need to feel this way, ever again. Do you hear me? *Ever* again.

A health care A-team is a group of doctors, specialists, and other health care providers who can help you handle tough times so you don't feel out of control, alone, lost, or desperate. Everyone who has a chronic health condition experiences flare-ups, and when those happen, your A-team can get you through them. Team members can communicate with each other and help determine a plan to get you to the other side. An A-team is crucial! It's a team you can count on during good times and bad so you don't go down the rabbit hole when a crisis hits.

Professionals who support you and make your health a priority are your safety net. Would you go skydiving without a parachute? I don't think so. That would be insane. So why would you try to manage your condition without the best team you can put together? If you don't, you'll be in a free fall with every health challenge.

The good news is that there are great doctors and other health care providers out there, and you can find them. Not only is getting an A-team together essential, but it's also completely possible!

My A-team includes my functional medicine practitioner (very important to find a go-to main doc), internist (here too), endocrinologist, chiropractor, motility specialist, acupuncturist, nutritionist, therapist, and life coach. I have worked hard to create relationships with each of these people. They are my parachutes if I have a flare-up or need a tune-up, and they are my team if I'm ever in a health crisis. These are the people who have shown they are able to step up to the plate.

When you get sick and feel desperate, it is hard to think beyond what is going to get you well immediately. The problem is, most of the time, not one doctor has every answer for you. In my experience, you have to try treatments and practitioners on for size and see what makes you feel good.

> A health care A-team is a group of doctors, specialists, and other health care providers who can help you handle tough times so you don't feel out of control, alone, lost, or desperate.

✓ EXERCISE *Your Dream Doc*

Instead of thinking about all of the wrong things you don't want in a doctor, let's figure out all of the things you do want in a doctor.

For this exercise, get out a sheet of paper or start a new page in your journal or use the dream doc checklist on this page. You're going to list everything you'd like your dream doctor—and any other health care worker—to be. This is your dream situation, so dream big! Go for it!

Here's one of my client's dream doctor list:

✓ Present

✓ Caring

✓ Kind

✓ Intuitive

✓ Confident

✓ Smart

✓ An expert in their field, but humble enough to keep learning

✓ On my team, willing to collaborate with other doctors and be a true partner with me on my quest toward health and healing

✓ Gives it to me straight

✓ Connects me with others if it will benefit my healing

✓ Simplifies the process by taking things slowly and steadily

✓ Practices what they preach

✓ Can admit when they don't have all the answers

✓ Pulls from all angles of medicine (Eastern and Western) and tailors a program to me

✓ Doesn't make me feel like a guinea pig

✓ Short waiting time for appointments

✓ Friendly and helpful staff (e.g., front desk staff, nurses, physician assistants)

✓ Good location for me

✓ Clean, brightly lit office; not depressing

✓ Takes my insurance

Once you finish your list, see how the qualities you listed match up with those of the health care providers you're seeing now. If anyone in your pool of health care providers doesn't have at least 85 percent of the qualities on your dream doctor list, it might be time to replace them, my friend.

My Dream Doc Checklist

My dream is for a health care system that easily allows a person's primary doctor to be in regular contact with everyone on that patient's A-team so they can all work together, or for a person to be able to go to a doctor's office that provides all of the things an A-team provides as one package. Medicine is certainly starting to move in that direction, but we aren't quite there yet. So for now, we have to create this for ourselves.

Healing that beautiful body takes time, and a quick pill isn't going to "fix" most chronic situations—or anything for that matter. For instance, if you're in the Chronic Condition Club, it's essential that you have a good functional medicine practitioner (or a solid internist) who gets you and what you are going through. This person can be your advocate and pull the threads of your spider web of doctors/healers/specialists/gurus together and communicate with them. The day I learned that an internist or functional medicine doctor could be the head of a team

There are great doctors and other health care providers out there, and you can find them.

of health care workers and could help coordinate my care, my life changed. Until then, I was running around like a chicken without a head, spinning in circles, trying to get through to people, and getting things faxed; managing my illness became managing my life. My illness was my life. Not anymore. This team effort lifts eighty pounds of stress right off your back. Your job is to get better, not to manage people.

Do your research. As I explained earlier in the chapter, you may have to make the rounds of specialists to rule out what is *not* wrong with you before you know what specialists you do need on your rock star A-team. See an immunologist if you are having immune system–related issues, a parasitologist to ensure you do not have parasites wreaking havoc on your systems, an endocrinologist to make sure your hormones aren't out of whack, and so on.

Once you have an A-team in place, you should create professional but personal relationships with each of them, and you should make sure they are accessible to you when you need them, for both short-term and long-term situations. If you put the time and care into forming these relationships, they will know you. They will know what kinds of situations come up for you, they know what kind of support you respond to, and they will be more willing to fit you in or work it out for you.

Also take the time to get to know the front-office people, the administrative staff, the physician assistants (PAs), and others who work at the offices of your A-team members. They can often get you in to see the doc fast, they may be able to talk to you on the phone to get you through certain situations, or they can help you with prescriptions or referrals.

The nurses especially are your best friends. Docs don't have time to talk to you about everything. A friendly nurse can help you with what you need, has direct communication with the doctor, and knows the ins and outs of the office. Make nice with the nurses! They can open doors—and get you through them.

Doc Talk 101: A Crash Course in Talking to Doctors

Even though my dad is a doctor, I didn't know much about effectively talking to doctors as a patient. It never occurred to me to ask him how to *talk* to a doctor when I first started my health journey. I assumed it was just like talking to regular people. So I sat down with my dad, and he gave me the 411 on doctorspeak, which is so important and something we all should know. He hooked me up. Now I can share it with you. Thanks, Dad!

Let's Get Organized

You should have a document on your computer that lists all the basic info for your A-team members. Load this document onto your smartphone so you can take it with you to every health care appointment you have. That way, it will be easily accessible if, let's say, you're planning to see a new specialist and need to fax something to your primary doc's office or you need two team members to communicate on an issue. You won't have to go home, get the necessary information, call the specialist's office back later, and wait on hold to terrible elevator music for ten minutes just to give them what they need. If you have everything right there on your phone, one, two, three, and you're done.

Your A-team list should include the name of each person and what they specialize in or are good at. The key is simplification.

- ▸ Name
- ▸ Specialty
- ▸ Address
- ▸ Phone number
- ▸ Fax number
- ▸ Email (if possible)
- ▸ Nurse's name
- ▸ Nurse's email

Initial Appointment

REHEARSE. Rule of thumb: when preparing for a doctor's appointment, pretend you have ten minutes to talk to the doctor. Practice ahead of time what you want to say to make sure you are concise during your appointment.

MAKE LISTS. Write down all of the topics, questions, and symptoms you want to discuss.

ELIMINATE REDUNDANCY. Make sure you're not telling the doctor the same thing two or three times. "I'm tired," "I'm fatigued," and "I'm sleepy" are all the same symptom. Be precise, and don't double back on symptoms. Apply the same guideline to your questions; make sure your list of questions doesn't include the same question worded multiple ways.

DECIDE WHAT IS MOST IMPORTANT. Ask yourself, what is your most important symptom? After that, move onto the next most important symptom. Apply the same guideline to your questions: rank them from most important to least important.

WRITE DOWN YOUR MEDICATIONS. Come prepared with a list of medicines you are taking now or have taken in the recent past. Say what you have been on

and why you were taken off other meds. Always consider supplements as medicines and put them on the list too. You can even consider giving a doctor a written list of what you're taking.

EXPLAIN YOUR DIET. Be prepared to talk about your diet and what and why you eat a certain way. Mention any special diets you've been on and how they made you feel. Make sure your symptoms list includes dramatic or unusual weight loss or gain.

BRING DOCUMENTATION. If you have any test results and lab reports, images, emergency room visit charts, or other medical reports from other health care pros, bring them to your first visit with a new doc. It may be helpful to send them in advance as well. Bring hard copies with you regardless.

STAY CALM AND MATTER-OF-FACT. As hard as it is for you to deal with chronic issues and scary symptoms, the more emotions you show, the harder it is for the doctor to deal with the medical problem in the short amount of time that you have.

Follow-Up Appointments

UPDATE YOUR LISTS. Start with the same lists of symptoms and questions you used at the first appointment. What has happened with that symptom between then and now? Is your top question the same as at the first visit, or has it changed?

FOCUS ON WHAT'S DIFFERENT AND NOT DIFFERENT. Talk about what has changed and what has stayed the same. Discuss what seems improved and what has not improved, if relevant.

Bills and Bureaucrats: How to Deal with Insurance Companies

Insurance sucks, especially when you have something complicated and chronic because most of the time you have to go out of network to see the best of the best docs. Our health care system is good at treating short-term problems, such as broken bones and infections. It needs to do a much better job managing chronic diseases. But until that happens, you have to deal with the insurance deck you're handed.

Average health care costs for someone who has one or more chronic conditions are five times greater than for someone without any chronic conditions. No wonder insurers will often try to find any way they can to not to reimburse you for a product or visit you have paid for!

Insurance companies can often seem like bullies when it comes to paying for treatments. Someone who feels fatigued and emotionally

"I was shocked with the multiple sclerosis (MS) diagnosis. Initially, I was prescribed Copaxone, which is injected. I had a real fear of needles and was resistant to the idea of giving myself injections. I researched alternatives and found the only oral medication for MS, Gilenya (formerly spelled *Gilenia,* generic name fingolimod) had just been approved by the FDA. It's more expensive than Copaxone, and my insurance company denied coverage. This didn't stop me; I decided to fight the insurance company.

I brought my case before a panel of people who decide whether to allow the coverage or not. I brought along my fiancé's mother, who is a lawyer; my father, also a lawyer; and a family friend who is a psychiatrist and could verify my fear of needles. I was very emotional when I told them all I had been through, with false diagnoses, the feeling of being out of control, my efforts to get pregnant. The insurance panel agreed with me and covered the oral med.

I am so glad I did not give up when I first got a denial from the insurance company. It pays to question, fight for what's right, and demand to be heard. If you have a forum, you should use it."

Lindsay White

and physically compromised is particularly vulnerable to these institutions and their rules, regulations, and incentives for employees not to approve payments. Sometimes I would feel too drained to lift my head off a pillow, let alone make a call to the insurance company. I would push off calling the company for weeks because I did not have the strength, emotionally or physically.

Here are some tips to help you deal.

GET CLEAR. Find out exactly what your insurance plan covers, including what docs and hospitals are covered and not covered. Determine how much out-of-network services will cost against your deductible, and plan to have out-of-network treatments as early in the year as possible. Deductibles restart each year, and starting treatments that will apply to your deductible will help you work off the deductible before you have to start all over with a new one when January rolls around. Starting early means you have a better chance of getting at least some out-of-network bills covered.

DELEGATE. If you have a complex case or have many questions or don't have the energy to handle it all, you can seek out a case manager at your insurer and make them part of your A-team. Yes, you have to ingratiate yourself so they are more prone to be sympathetic and helpful. Talk to the same person every time so you do not have to explain yourself constantly.

TIME IT. If you are sick at the end of December (when your insurance cycle ends), try to wait until January to get and submit bills so they are dated January (when your new insurance cycle begins). That way you will get a whole year to work off the deductible and get post-dated deductible bills paid. If you start submitting bills in November (and I understand you may have to), you will likely not meet that year's deductible before starting all over with the full deductible in January.

STAND UP. Learn the process for challenging your insurance company's decision to decline to cover certain procedures or drugs. You do have the right to challenge decisions and resubmit claims. It takes energy, but it's possible and can lead to a favorable change of mind on the insurer's part.

▼ ▼ ▼

Take a moment to think about how you are set up currently and how you can shift your health game. You are in control. Create your team. Write down what you want to change. Make it a priority to make those changes reality.

5

Wellness Work 101

During my healing crisis, I felt like crap. This lasted for a long time and I eventually decided I didn't want to feel that way anymore. So I put my thinking-smart cap on and came to realize that complementary healing modalities could be very powerful for me. As a result, along my windy road toward healing, I've had many wellness therapies and treatments that have helped me, so much so that some of the practitioners are on my A-team. What I know for sure is this: there are treatments and healers who can help your body feel better and lift it into a more elevated state than it is currently in. While the traditional docs do their thang, your tribe of wellness workers and alternative treatments can support your body and soul on its healing journey. They can improve the quality of your life and add some fuel to your tank. It is up to you to figure out who and what works for you. Creating a support system and adding these practitioners to your A-team is super important for your healing. Why shouldn't you have this? You are so worth it.

There's absolutely nothing wrong with exploring complementary treatments that may help you and that have real and proven health benefits. The relationship you have with yourself and how you treat yourself is crucial to healing. Incorporating what feels right for you from this section can bring you back to your heart center, and to the relationship you have with your body, so that you can heal.

I have been to what seems like one thousand wellness workers. Okay, that's an exaggeration. But I've definitely made the rounds so that you don't have to. What follows is my list of wellness work that I find to be beneficial. It's not a comprehensive guide to every form of wellness work. If you discover a practice that's not on this list, by all means try it out. If it helps you, keep going; if not, move on. Any of the complementary services I describe here can support your well-being, reduce your stress levels, augment your healing, and enhance your quality of life.

Acupuncture

There were times when I would go see an acupuncturist several times a week for both acupuncture and cupping. First and foremost, it helped relax and center me more than any other treatment in the thick of my healing crisis. When I was detoxing from heavy metal issues, I found acupuncture to be particularly helpful in terms of not only relaxation, but also in getting my blood circulating and moving toxins out of my system. Look for an acupuncturist who is familiar with people who have chronic issues.

Cupping helps move stagnation in the blood and get the blood flowing. Acupuncture is amazingly helpful from something as simple as getting a cold to drain out of your body to getting stagnant energy moving through your body if you are chronically sick. Plus, an acupuncture treatment feels like taking a ride on the peace train, and who doesn't want to go on that ride?

Chiropractic

It wasn't until I added a type of chiropractic work called Sacro Occipital Technique (SOT) into my regular routine that I started to feel essentially pain-free. SOT work gave me a good reference point for pain and discomfort in my body. I then started to remember what it felt like for my muscular-skeletal system to be in total alignment—something I hadn't felt since before my back pain began at age fourteen.

Having my spine and neuromuscular system in alignment deeply helped me re-identify with my body as my home, and not just some thing I was living in that wasn't working well. When these foundational parts of the body are in proper alignment, your entire physical system is set up to succeed. Chiropractic care makes me feel calmer, stronger, more awake, and more in tune with what my body is trying to tell me. I now am able to reference what being in alignment feels like, and it feels pretty amazing, so when something feels off, I am better able to tune in to what my body is trying to tell me. Chiropractic care, particularly SOT, is a staple in my healing journey.

Craniosacral Therapy

I tried craniosacral therapy when I took the plunge into my alternative-healing party. I found it to be incredibly relaxing. Every part of us is interconnected, so when one area of the body is relaxed, another responds to that. Craniosacral therapy is a form of bodywork. Practitioners use therapeutic touch on your head, spine, and pelvis to regulate the flow of cerebrospinal fluid through the spine and to manipulate the synarthrodial joints of the cranium. How's that for a tongue twister? Seriously, it's divine. It can definitely relieve anxiety and stress, and is extremely relaxing when done by an experienced person with an experienced touch.

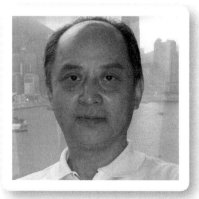

Tsoi Nam Chan, DTCM

Tsoi Nam Chan is a doctor of traditional Chinese medicine (TCM), naturopath, and iridologist. He has been practicing for over thirty-seven years in the United States. He was trained in China and has done extensive research with the Chinese Health Department in head acupuncture (acupuncture for conditions such as stroke, paralysis, and coma). He has integrated Western holistic medicine with his TCM background, creating a more effective combination of healing arts to provide patients with the highest level of care. He is considered one of the leading authorities of TCM.

Here, Tsoi Nam Chan shares the value of acupuncture and cupping for those with chronic conditions.

Acupuncture involves stimulating anatomical locations on the skin using a variety of techniques. Thin, solid, metallic needles are commonly used; they are manipulated manually or by electrical stimulation. Acupuncture has been used for over 2,500 years in China and is now used all over the world to treat people's illnesses, not just their symptoms. The reason it still exists is that it works. Since 1996, the U.S. Food and Drug Administration (FDA) has classified acupuncture needles as medical devices for "general use" by trained professionals.

Most major hospitals, including Memorial Sloan Kettering, Johns Hopkins, and New York Hospital, now have acupuncture departments. More medical doctors, including neurologists, anesthesiologists, and specialists in physical medicine, are becoming trained in acupuncture.

Acupuncture is important to a person with a chronic health condition. There are fourteen major energy channels, called *Jingmais,* that flow through the human body, including through the head, arms, hands, legs, feet, and torso. These Jingmais connect all the internal organs. A subtle energy called *Qi* (pronounced *chee*) circulates via the Jingmais to all parts of the body, even the most remote cells. Qi is the vital force, the presence of which separates the living from the dead. Its balanced and unimpeded flow is critical to sound health. Any misdirection, blockage, ▶

▶ or other derangement of the amount, flow, or balance of Qi may result in pain, dysfunction, and ill health. The needles used in acupuncture are placed in very specific points (there are over two thousand points!) along your body to coordinate with your energy channels, thus helping to re-balance your system by strengthening weaknesses and balancing excesses of energy.

Acupuncture helps restore the normal balance and flow of Qi so organs and bodily systems can work together in harmony, as intended. This sets the stage for the body to repair itself and maintain its own health without drugs. Acupuncture has been used to treat an array of ailments, ranging from headaches and chemotherapy-induced nausea, to joint pain and postoperative pain. In fact, the American College of Rheumatology, a major organization for medical professionals who treat arthritis and other musculoskeletal diseases, endorses the use of acupuncture for chronic pain.

Cupping is a related therapeutic technique in which glass, bamboo, or ceramic cups are applied to the body with a vacuum pump or heat. For example, in the heating method, a burning, alcohol-soaked cotton ball is waved inside the cup in order to create the needed vacuum. It feels as if the cup is pulling onto the skin. The cups are placed mainly over acupuncture points or locations experiencing pain or tension and left there for five to ten minutes. To remove the cups, the skin next to the opening of the cup is pressed, allowing air to seep in to detach the cup.

Cupping is based on the belief that blood stagnation in the muscles and body is the cause of illnesses and pain. Circulation improves with the technique. The red or purple marks left after treatment helps a cupping practitioner see where blood is circulating well and where it is not; a darker mark would indicate poor circulation, and, upon subsequent visits, lighter marks would indicate improvement. Typically, cupping has been practiced to stimulate blood flow, loosen tight muscles, manage pain, and strip toxins from the body.

Remember that there are different types of medical systems, Eastern and Western. However, all humans are the same earth beings, and there is no such a thing as East and West in terms of illness. ■

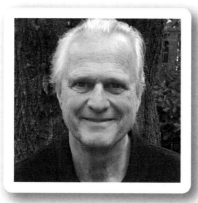

Michael J. Cindrich, DC, DICS

Michael J. Cindrich is a doctor of chiropractic (DC). He is a member of the American Chiropractic Association (ACA), the New York State Chiropractic Association (NYSCA), and the Sacro Occipital Research Society International (SORSI). Dr. Cindrich holds basic and advanced certifications in Sacro Occipital Technic (SOT), as well as craniopathy, in which he holds a diplomate degree. He is also an ACA-certified chiropractic sports physician (CCSP). He has written and presented numerous papers about his specialties and has had over twenty years of extensive teaching experience within the chiropractic profession.

Here Dr. Cindrich shares some basic information about chiropractic care and SOT and how they can help alleviate symptoms of chronic conditions.

The World Health Organization defines *health* as "[t]he state of complete physical, mental, and social well-being and not merely the absence of disease or infirmity." Chiropractic is a natural healing art. It is a drug-free, hands-on approach to health used to help restore the body's natural vigor and vitality. Chiropractic care is so important in keeping optimum nerve flow to fortify a strong immune defense system and maintain vibrant good health. In fact, the word *chiropractic* derives from the Greek and means "by hand." General hands-on chiropractic works very well for very many people. "Miracles" occur all the time in chiropractic offices all over the world.

I use a chiropractic method called Sacro Occipital Technic, or SOT. Major Bertrand DeJarnette, a chiropractor, osteopath, and engineer, as well as a visionary genius, first originated the work back in the 1920s. He then developed his work and taught it around the world until just before his passing in 1992. He preferred to use the word *technic,* an engineering term, over *technique.* SOT is now a registered trademark of SORSI, a research and teaching organization founded by DeJarnette.

SOT is a system of analysis and adjusting the body that is based upon an indicator system. In other words, the innate intelligence of the body will give the practitioner a reliable, scientifically sound method of ascertaining which area of the cranium, spinal column, pelvis, extremity, or soft tissue needs ▶

adjusting, and then will often give immediate feedback as to how well that adjustment has been accepted by the body. This takes a lot of stress off of the doctor. We just follow the directives of the body as we try to assist it in restoring its vital integrity. ■

Massage Therapy

Who doesn't love a good rub down? If you have a chronic illness, you likely feel weak, tired, and achy often. Am I right? Having someone massage your sore muscles and bring some attention and love to the sore parts of your body simply feels like such a great treat, and it helps you relax. I particularly recommend it late in the day before you go to slumber town. Other than the warm hug or gentle touch of a loved one, a massage has to be the ultimate healing human touch.

There are so many different kinds of massage—Swedish, deep tissue, Shiatsu, and so on—that finding the one you like best may take time. Some people like very deep, strong massages, while others like a lighter touch.

Massage can alleviate low-back pain and improve range of motion. It enhances immunity by stimulating the lymphatic system—the body's natural defense system. It can help get rid of muscle knots in your neck, legs, back, and shoulders. It promotes tissue regeneration, which over time can reduce scar tissue and stretch marks. Well-executed massage pumps oxygen and nutrients into tissues and vital organs, and it improves circulation. It also releases endorphins—amino acids that work as the body's natural painkillers and mood lifters.

Reflexology

Reflexology is a type of bodywork that focuses on the feet, based on the theory that there are reflex areas on the feet that correspond to specific organs, glands, and other parts of the body. According to the reflexology theory, every part of our body has a correlating point on the feet. For instance, the tips of the toes reflect the head; the heart and chest are reflected around the ball of the foot; the liver, pancreas, and kidney correspond with points in the arch of the foot; and the lower back and intestines are represented in an area toward the heel. Reflexology can help relieve stress, tension headaches, arthritis, digestive issues, and sleep problems. It promotes relaxation, improves circulation, reduces pain, and encourages overall healing.

Most people find reflexology for the most part to be very relaxing, and many people's bodies respond really well to it. While a reflexologist works only with your feet, you actually do feel the effects in your entire body, amazing as that sounds. They use brisk hand movements to warm up your feet, and then move seamlessly into a deep tissue foot massage, pinpointing areas of the feet where they feel you need the most help. Divine!

The more in tune with my body I have gotten, the more I have seen the benefits of reflexology. It is amazing that if a part of your body aches, you can look at a reflexology map of your foot and match a specific place on your foot to the body area you struggle with. How cool is that? When you are in the CC Club, and especially if you have areas of your body that need a little TLC, it can be very helpful to have a reflexologist focus on the areas of your feet that directly correspond to the part of the body affected by the ailment or illness you are dealing with. By targeting a specific area of the body directly, reflexology can speed up relief to the part of the body that is struggling. Plus, who doesn't love a deep, luxurious foot rub? *Just sayin'.*

Colon Hydrotherapy

Colon hydrotherapy has greatly helped me because of my motility disorder. In fact, it had such an important effect on my quality of life that I became a practitioner in order to become an expert on my condition and to fully understand why detoxification is so

The Healing Power of Touch

Have you ever noticed that when someone reaches out to touch you during a conversation, especially a difficult one, their touch softens the situation, and you feel more cared for or listened to? When you're under the weather, a hug or a back rub from a loved one seems to have restorative powers, doesn't it? Well, there's a reason for that. When another person touches you, the signals sent to your brain translate into feelings of security, happiness, and comfort. Touch also promotes trust and generosity between people.

One of the first studies that demonstrated the incredible healing power of human touch was done during WWII. Dr. René Spitz noted that babies who were hugged, held, and cuddled thrived and grew better than those who were not, despite receiving the same nutrition and health care.[1] After extensive study years later, the American psychologist Harry Harlow determined that human touch is essential if people are going to thrive and heal.[2] Another study done at Brigham Young University found that the test group who had experienced supportive touch showed lower blood pressure levels and higher natural levels of oxytocin.[3]

important for the body, especially when it's in a compromised state. If you have a traffic jam all the way up the George Washington Bridge, how can you possibly go full speed forward? You can't, so when you're that backed up, there is pressure and stress on every single part of your body and every organ, tissue, and cell in it. It is crucial to keep the pathways clear so you can properly detoxify and keep internal stress at bay. Digestive issues are no joke, and boy are they a drag to deal with. Whether you're dealing with something like my condition (slow-transit constipation), irritable bowel syndrome (IBS), or other chronic intestinal conditions, or even just a minor feeling of constipation, this work can help your large intestine and give your entire body a reboot when it comes to your elimination station.

Other Wellness Therapies

All of the wellness therapies I've described so far are administered by practitioners. I can also testify to the good effects of two other complementary therapies: flotation tank therapy and infrared sauna therapy.

Flotation Tank Therapy

Flotation tanks are large soundproof pods that contain water with a high density of Epsom salt. So, yeah, a session is like an uber-Epsom-salt bath—the best one you've ever had. The sensory deprivation of the tank puts your body naturally into the state you were in in the womb.

Flotation tank therapy can help alleviate stress, depression, insomnia, anxiety, arthritis, and chronic pain. Personally, I have experienced immediate tension relief and pain relief with flotation tank therapy. In fact, you can experience even more benefits with each session as you get into the flow of the therapy and allow yourself to relax as soon as you get into the tank. You can go into a deep meditative state almost immediately.

Flotation tank therapy literally puts your body in a state of bliss within seconds. It takes all of the weight off and discomfort out of your body, your joints, and your muscles. It supports your body in reaching a state of relaxation that is as deep as the deepest form of sleep. It also takes away all sensory distractions, and you are just alone with your body and your breath in a totally comfortable and relaxed setting. Not every city and town offers flotation tanks, but if you ever have a chance to try it, I recommend it highly, especially if you have chronic conditions related to stress and depression, arthritis or joint pain, or problems sleeping. The more you can relax your body, the easier it will be to heal. If I haven't convinced you yet, the New England Patriots and many other professional teams have them in their training facilities. Got ya!

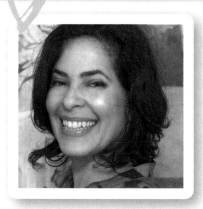

Cindy Suarez, LE, CCH

Cindy Suarez is the cofounder of DTX: Cellular Evolution in New York City, a full-service colon therapy clinic. She is a licensed esthetician and a certified colon hydrotherapist.

Here, Cindy discusses the benefits of colon therapy.

Simply put, colon hydrotherapy is bathing the large intestine. Through the use of warm water, we assist the large intestine in loosening and flushing gasses and waste that are on their way out, but at times hang out a little too long and accumulate in the system.

Some people think if the colon is full, we just empty it, and that's all colon therapy is about. Colon therapy does so much more. What happens when you empty the colon is that you send a message on a deeper level throughout your body to all of your cells. Emptying the colon gives your body a chance to heal and release toxins at the cellular level. When you do that, everything starts to heal. The benefits from cleansing the colon can affect your ears, that little eye infection, acne, high blood pressure, inflammation—a lot of symptoms can be cleared from the body through this one tool.

We have an elimination system for a reason, and that reason is to help us get rid of what we don't need. The reason you want to flush your system with a colonic today is that we are not living in natural times anymore. We live in cities. We live under stress. We live in compromised conditions—air quality, water quality, food quality. It's like ▶

▶ a layer cake, which has become heavier with pollutants. Unless you eliminate three or four times a day, you are allowing toxins to accumulate in your tissues. Everything that you put on your skin, everything you breathe, and everything you ingest goes right into your system. That is a lot of intake. When you clear the elimination system and when you eat well, you start making space in your digestive system / large intestine so that the small intestine and the stomach acids can start healing.

Colonics do not create dependency. That is a myth. If anything, they help people establish more freedom. Colon therapy is like physical therapy; do you think that you will not be able to use that ankle again or that limb if you do not have help? No, it gets stronger. The colon is a muscle. It is also an organ, but it is a muscle, and it can be very strong. We just need to give it the chance. During a colonic, you empty the colon and relieve it of the burden of holding on to extra waste and air. You are giving it a bit of a workout and helping your colon become more efficient. ■

Infrared Sauna Therapy

An infrared sauna is a great way to get the benefits of penetrating heat, allowing it to reach into your body to stimulate healthy sweating. An infrared sauna differs from a traditional sauna because it raises your core body temperature, thus helping you sweat more quickly and more profusely. This deep-down heat is very soothing to joints and muscles. When your body heats up, it generates more white blood cells, which strengthens your immune system. As you sweat, you begin to breathe faster, your heart works a bit harder, your circulation improves, and your metabolism accelerates in a concerted effort to resume your normal body temperature.

Since your circulation is increased during sweating, many toxins and impurities are able to exit your body by way of your open skin pores. Your skin is your body's largest organ, and it benefits big time from infrared sauna sweating.

Find the Right People and Services

Make sure that the service providers you choose are the best you can find—the all-stars of their league. Don't just walk into someone's office straight from a Google search because you were being lazy and theirs was the first name you saw. Your bod is super sensitive. When you are in the CC Club, people with experience and good vibrations matter. We need people who have seen and treated patients like us, who have been around the block long enough that they feel comfortable taking care of us with an open mind, and who have a real presence and a whole lotta heart.

How do you find these magical people that are just the right fit for you? For me, it became easier to find the right wellness workers for my A-team once I had the docs and other health care provider members in place. Your medical A-team is the best place to start when looking for alternative practitioners because they usually are hooked into the entire health care community. If they don't have suggestions, ask trusted friends or colleagues. Ideally, you want someone who has come highly recommended by someone you trust. No time to waste! While you are trying wellness workers on for size, make sure that they are tender, present, and deserving of your coming for a service. I went to ten acupuncturists before I found the right one. That isn't a joke. I love me some acupuncture, so I was on a big, bad mission to find the best one for *me*. One seemed way too timid and almost afraid of my condition (yeah, that makes me feel really relaxed); I swear she was practically shivering while writing down my medical history. Another talked to me throughout the whole entire treatment as if I was her best girlfriend, even though I didn't respond once and, quite

The Big Quit: Do I Need This?

As you become more tuned in to your body and feelings, you also will have a lot of clarity about what is working and what isn't. If you are in a sea of treatments, as I was, check in with yourself to see if what you are doing is still serving you. If it is, keep it going; if it isn't, time to let it go. Same goes for the docs. The Big Quit should not be a big deal. Make a list of all the wellness workers you're seeing and all the alternative therapies you're doing now. For each one, answer the following five questions honestly. If you answer yes to most of the questions, continue the service. But if you answer no to most of them, it may be high time for the Big Quit.

▸ Do I look forward to my appointments?

▸ Am I happy going into the therapy?

▸ Do I make the next appointment eagerly?

▸ Do I feel noticeably better after the therapy or service?

▸ Do I value this service more than something else I could be doing at the same time?

You should leave from any wellness treatment feeling more balanced, stronger, peaceful, and more centered than you did before you came in.

frankly, just wanted to chill out. Another one's office just felt off to me; I didn't like the energy immediately upon entering, and things did not improve the longer I stayed. Another acupuncturist's office smelled like the right kind of incense, had just the right Enya tunes playing, and had just the right number of spiritual books stacked up in the waiting room, but she didn't have the professional chops to back up her rad office. So although I felt peaceful in the space, I didn't leave feeling peaceful in my body. (See? I really wasn't joking when I said I have done everything so you don't have to.)

When you find the right practitioner, you will know, my sweet friend. You will feel taken care of. You will know if the person feels right and the treatment is helpful and does what it is supposed to do. When you make a commitment to an alternative treatment and practitioner, a deep dive is in order. Tell them all about your health journey, show

them your relevant medical records, and share your vulnerable truth with them.

You should leave from any wellness treatment—whether it's acupuncture, a massage, or any other type of bodywork—feeling more balanced, stronger, peaceful, and more centered than you did before you came in. You should feel at home in your body. You should feel much more able to conquer your day and do the little things you usually feel you can't, and have a sense of support that you didn't have before you went in.

Quality not Quantity

Most caregivers, conventional and alternative, believe they can help you heal, but the bottom line is not all of them can help *you*. You have to figure out which wellness treatments and workers truly serve you and eliminate who and what doesn't because running from one treatment and therapy to another can be expensive and exhausting. At one point I was doing vitamin shots and IVs every day, in every place on my bod, to help my nutrient deficiencies. I was running to acupuncture, and then across town to the colon therapist, and then downtown to the chiropractor, and then back uptown to a conventional doctor again, and then to the lab all the way across town to get my blood work done, and then home to do a stool test. No joke. I was totally wiped out. In fact, I feel drained just writing about it.

I literally just kept running. This, my friends, is the flight version of the fight-or-flight response—or at least the way it presented itself in me. I was like a speeding train with no stop in sight, and I didn't even realize it because I was so desperate to find a solution immediately.

When one doctor said to me, "Well, we could give this thing a shot. Maybe that will work. Who knows?" my head snapped back. I thought to myself, "Huh? *Maybe* that will work? *Who knows?*"

The doctor's shot-in-the-dark uncertainty made me feel like a lab rat or a voodoo doll. And my *body* very clearly said to my *mind,* "That's it. Mama needs a break. I'm out."

First, my bod and I went on strike. We slept—and slept and slept and slept. Next, I paused—something I had truly never done up until that point. (In fact, if I hadn't had that experience with the doctor, I would still be speeding on through life.) When I hit the pause button, I started evaluating what services and therapies were actually helping and serving me and which ones were not. I had added so many potions to the pot that it had become a witch's cauldron. For two months after my colon therapist closed her office and after surviving the break away from Dr. Cure-All, I stopped every other treatment I was doing, except the readjustment of my thyroid meds. It was only then that I could clear my head and choose wisely among the many treatments available.

If you are having too many treatments and therapies, you might forget what's what and what is truly serving you best. Remember, the point of all of these treatments is to feel better, not more depleted. Make sure you are tuning in to what feels right for you now—not what felt right a week ago, not what will feel right a month in the future, but what feels right here, right now. Keep it simple.

6

Food Fabulous Food!

I love to eat great food and have a good time doing it. Always have. That's still the case, I'm happy to say. But I have been on a wild food journey for as long as I can remember. It was a long time before I learned to have a positive, *healthy*, loving relationship with food because I didn't know that what I put in my mouth had a direct correlation with my health. Frozen dinners and boxed or canned convenience products filled with chemicals and sold as "healthy" stocked my family's fridge and pantry. As a kid, I remember many afternoons sitting on the floor of the basement family room, eating a Costco-sized case of Fruit Gushers as a mid-morning snack. Later, I'd have a pizza bagel for lunch.

By the time I got to college, my morning routine had to include a *venti* coffee with two extra shots if I wanted to function on the most basic level. I thought it was completely normal for a typical college girl on the go to chug that much caffeine in order to simply wake up. After graduating, I worked as a cocktail waitress to supplement my income as an actress. Those of you who are in the

hospitality industry know this can be a toxic work environment. You're so tired when your shift is over, all you want to do is knock back a short one, wolf down some cheese fries, and crawl into bed. Not to mention that, surprise, surprise, when you work in a bar, drinking is cheap and easy. It also leads to hangovers, dry skin, and raccoon eyes. Not exactly an ashram of healthy livin'. You feel me?

In 2008, I had my wake-up call. One morning, I was feeling more exhausted and anxious than usual. The huge dark circles under my eyes, brittle hair, and adult acne were bad enough; I was heavier than I liked, and I was more fatigued than I had ever felt in my life. I was spent. A good look in the mirror showed me someone whom I wasn't sure I liked. Right then and there I made a decision never to look and feel that way again. I was sick and tired of feeling sick, tired, and pained.

I started a personal food revolution, reading everything I could get my hands on about nutrition and the connection between food and disease, among other topics. It blew my mind to learn that the traditional government-sponsored food pyramid, heavily influenced by various food lobbies, and heavy with wheat, meat, and dairy products, wasn't actually doing me any good. This realization made me feel vulnerable and emotional as it was *everything* I was raised eating. A food pyramid with veggies on the bottom, instead of wheat- and grain-based carbs, and with meat and dairy at the very top, is so much healthier.

It is so important to listen to your body and find out exactly what it wants.

After this life-altering experience, I truly understood the importance of proper nourishment and that what I put into my body means everything when it comes to my health. It is so important to listen to your body and find out exactly what it wants. Unfortunately, too many of us eat what is aptly named SAD: the standard American diet. The SAD is *no bueno* mostly because processed carbs (cereals, crackers, chips, breads, pasta, cookies, cakes) dominate it and are followed by genetically modified, hormone- and antibiotic-stuffed, processed meat products (yum!), with a few fruits and

veggies sprinkled in. Yup, even that expensive artisanal brie and turkey sandwich on sourdough, labeled "healthy choice," is crap.

The SAD is nutrient light and low in basic vitamins, minerals, fiber, phytonutrients, amino acids, and other good stuff that enables us to glow from the inside out. But it is high in many other things: hydrogenated oil, high-fructose corn syrup, phytic acid, acrylamide, sodium nitrate, genetically modified bits and pieces, and monosodium glutamate (MSG). Your body doesn't need, doesn't want, can't use, and doesn't know what to do with this junk.

After my research blitz, I slowed my roll on the huge sources of gluten and dairy that had become staples in my diet. Green juices and more veggies, including large, organic salads, became part of my daily routine. With time I started to function, feel, and look so much better. *Finally,* I was starting to come to a place of balance and peace in my body.

Then I went to Israel, and my newfound awesome lifestyle was abandoned. You could have called me gluten girl because I was eating a lot of it in the form of pita bread accompanied by falafel and hummus. At this point I was still unaware that I had celiac disease. So it was the perfect storm; my whole physical universe exploded. My back was on fire again. All my previous symptoms returned with a vengeance, and new ones joined in, including those from a parasite who set up shop in my tummy and crashed the party, bringing along its entire family.

When I said in chapter 1 that I gained thirty pounds in thirty days (that's more than six liters of water!), my hair fell out in clumps, and my limbs felt like they were aching off, I wasn't kidding. When I got back home, I tried getting back to my healthy eating routine. Unfortunately, my health continued to spiral out of control. I could not keep food down or go to the bathroom. After my trip abroad, my gastric system went haywire, and my large and small intestines were failing me. The only things I could keep down were juices, protein shakes, green smoothies, and broth. I lived on those foods for more than a year while I tried to figure out why I was having an intestinal shutdown.

Eventually, I was diagnosed with celiac disease. That, combined with the parasite infection and problems with my thyroid, produced a brilliant trifecta that my GI system has yet to fully recover from. The painkillers I'd taken throughout my childhood and into my college years, plus an intense bout of mononucleosis I'd had in college, only added to everything causing my body to strike out. Two days after I ditched gluten at the door, my back stopped hurting, and it's never given me problems since. Now I know how important food is for my health and well-being. Eating foods that support my health is the bedrock of all my self-care.

> The moment we start nourishing our precious bodies with the best ingredients, a powerful, positive shift in our health and well-being takes place.

For me, eating healthfully isn't a luxury; it's a life-saving necessity.

As a society, we have completely lost the connections between food and fuel, and food and wellness. We need to understand *why* a diet dominated by meat, wheat, dairy, and sugar is so problematic for health. Americans didn't always eat the SAD way. Let's go back to a time when things were happier, simpler, and less processed. There was life before high-fructose corn syrup, triple caramel lattes, and red dye number one. And it was the good life! Once upon a time it was the norm for people to make simple, delicious food from real, seasonal ingredients. The moment we start nourishing our precious bodies with the best ingredients, a powerful, positive shift in our health and well-being takes place. So bye-bye Burger King, Wendy, and Ronald and *helloooo* spinach, carrots, kale, and cucumbers!

"The body is an amazing creation, and it wants to support you. But when you live out of alignment with what your body needs to feel good, it has problems keeping up. If you are open to change and look at gluten-free living as an adventure and an experiment, it helps you see the possibilities instead of the restrictions. It's not about what you can't eat; it's about what you *can* eat. I can find plenty of food I can eat and so many delicious ways to prepare it. You have permission to try new foods, and you have permission to spit 'em out and try again if you don't like 'em!"

Jennifer Fugo

End the Acid Trip: The Alkaline Factor

Bottom line: everything you put into your body affects it. In the Chronic Condition Club, we need to do everything we can to support our bodies in terms of a healthy lifestyle, and food plays a huge part in this effort. Since a lot of us (myself included) have become accustomed to eating convenience foods on the fly, we've ended up taking a very bad acid trip.

Our body's alkaline and acid balance, also known as pH, has a direct effect on our health and well-being. Everything we eat and drink has an effect—positive, negative, or neutral—on our normal pH. You don't need to know the entire scientific explanation of pH, but some background is helpful. Water has a neutral pH of 7. Blood has a pH of 7.35 to 7.45, which is slightly alkaline. Your bod loves being slightly alkaline and does its thing to keep it that way. Your internal fluids and tissues do not stay in a set state of acidity or alkalinity, but instead fluctuate as the body strives toward finding the perfect balance. If you keep putting your body on an acid trip by way of too much dairy, burgers, and chicken nuggets, it finds it difficult to maintain the perfect pH balance. A dangerous imbalance sets in, and the body must spend its time and energy dealing with the resulting stress and inflammation.

Inflammation is a bitch out of hell. Inflammation (that fucker) is oftentimes the root cause, or one of them, of our health issues, and most likely a huge underlying reason 50 percent of Americans have a chronic disease. A state of chronic inflammation, or the

Our body's alkaline and acid balance, also known as pH, has a direct effect on our health and well-being.

By reducing the amount of the acidity-promoting foods we eat, we reduce inflammation in our body.

nonstop production of immune cells, can do permanent damage to our bodies and lead to all sorts of ugliness, like cancer, heart disease, arthritis, kidney stones (ouch!), and, yeah, you guessed it, a host of other chronic health conditions. If the body reaches an acidic state, it is basically sending an invitation to all things bad to come on in and trash the place.

But here is the good news: by reducing the amount of the acidity-promoting foods we eat, we reduce inflammation in our body.

The key to reducing acidity is boosting alkaline levels. Alkalinity is the by-product of digesting dark green vegetables, sea algae, and other plant foods. These beautiful foods are the front line in the war against inflammation. The chlorophyll found in green plants (the stuff that's responsible for their remarkable emerald color) has amazing antioxidant, anti-inflammatory, and wound-healing properties. It delivers magnesium and helps the blood carry much-needed oxygen to our cells and tissues. Oh yeah, it has vitamins too, including A, C, and E.

Alkaline-rich foods alleviate serious stress in the body by countering inflammation. An alkaline diet can result in increased stamina and strength, a stronger immune system, better energy, and a million other glowy things! Its real super power (as if that wasn't enough)? It's a gangster against free radicals, the shit that damages our cells. It helps neutralize them—zap! As result, we look, feel, and function better.

Giving your body lots of veggies and plant-based foods is like giving it a pair of powerful boxing gloves that can combat and prevent a ton of health issues.

A plant-centric diet is the way to go if you want to really go green. Giving your body lots of veggies and plant-based foods is like giving it a pair of powerful boxing gloves that can combat and prevent a ton of health issues. So give produce the starring role it deserves in your diet. Upping the alkalinity factor of our diets floods our grateful insides with the good stuff it craves. There's no excuse *not* to choose nutrient-dense, fresh, whole delicious foods flooded with the amino acids, enzymes, vitamins, and minerals necessary to help our bodies and minds thrive. Another great benefit of many alkaline foods, fresh produce specifically, is that they contain plenty of fiber, which helps us feel full and eliminate easily.

Veggies and especially leafy and cruciferous greens (like good ol' kale) are bursting with phytochemicals or phytonutrients. There are more than twenty-five thousand phytonutrients in plants, and scientists have just scratched the surface of those that are important for humans. In nature, out in the garden, these warriors protect plants from germs, fungi, and bugs, and a lot of research says they do the same thing for us: help us prevent disease and keep our insides running smoothly.

The plate isn't the only powerful way to flood your body with alkalinity. A daily green juice, green smoothie, or shot of wheatgrass is a great way to power your day. Drinking a fresh-made juice with spinach, kale, and a small green apple or a green smoothie is a much better alternative to having coffee with sugar and half-and-half and a donut for breakfast. A leafy green salad (the darker the leaves, the better) with or *for* dinner is another simple way to keep your machine running lean, clean, and mean.

That's not to say you can't have acidic foods ever again. Many whole foods, like beans and grains, are slightly acidic. Besides, who says we can't have a cappuccino (with almond milk) or a chocolate chip cookie on the rare occasion? Not this girl. So cool it. I am not telling you to abandon all the foods you love, ditch your canned tuna completely, and become a 300 percent raw vegan. What I *am* saying is to take the wheat-meat-dairy trifecta down about ten notches, eliminating it as much as possible. Get rid of junk food, especially the sugar. Sugar is insidious, so you have to be a detective to find all the places it hides.

Cozy Up to Your Kitchen

The best way to start eating yourself healthy is to get rid of foods that don't serve your body. Don't worry: I also give you a list of great goodies that should replace the scary stuff.

Ditch the Debris

Patrol that pantry! You're on duty. Toss! Here's a list of junky-junk to get rid of:

- Anything with a shelf life the same age as you (duh).

- All things processed and white have got to go. Yup, that means white rice, white potatoes, white sugar, and white bread.

- Anything with gluten. Whether you're gluten sensitive or not, gluten is an inflammatory food, and it's not good for a body that is compromised by a chronic condition. Plus, we don't need gluten to survive and thrive. It's unnecessary nutritionally. So we want to straight up ditch the gluten.

- Any food product with more than ten ingredients, including "preservatives" and "stabilizers" and "natural flavoring." Or anything you don't understand and can barely read or pronounce.

- Any food with artificial colors, dyes, or flavors; or foods with artificial fat and sugar replacements.

- Soda.

- Corn and corn-based products, including corn syrup (not easy on our bellies).

- Animal products that are not from organic, sustainable sources.

- All refined-sugar products.

- Inflammatory foods: dairy (milk, cheese, butter, yogurt), corn, soy, and nightshades (tomatoes, bell peppers, white potatoes, eggplant).

- Fruit high in sugar (cherries, bananas, figs, and all dried fruit).

The Perfect Plate

To create a beautiful plate, make it 75 percent veggie, with the 25 percent balance coming from protein (a serving of protein in the size of your palm) and healthy fats.

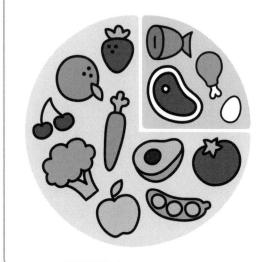

Get Down and Dirty

A fun and social way to start embracing veggies, and a good way to nudge your creative side into action and get that cute butt of yours into the kitchen, is to get up close and personal with produce. Get your fingernails dirty! Go to your local farmer's market and look, touch, smell, and sample what's available (with permission, of course!). Talk to the farmers about what they grow and how to prepare it. Bring a friend and make it an occasion. Talk to other shoppers. Food lovers and farmers love to share information.

Get adventurous and try something you've never had, like zucchini flowers, fiddlehead ferns, or mustard greens. Go at the end of the day, and you might score a box of carrots or a few heads of lettuce at bargain basement prices. Juice 'em up if you can't use 'em up in a salad.

Or how about digging around in some dirt in your own backyard? Maybe start a little victory garden—victory over chronic disease—by planting some super-easy-to-grow lettuce, cucumber, squash, and green beans. When you have seasonal veggies, you are more likely to want to incorporate them into the kitchen and get connected to food. Fuel, flavor, *and* fun! Check!

Make Your Kitchen Glow with These Nutrition Warriors

Once you have given all of those bad things the boot, like a bad boyfriend and his smelly leather jacket, you gotta stock up on the gems and jewels of the food world. If your cupboards are bare, you'll be calling Dial-a-Pizza at midnight. Eek! Let's go shopping:

VEGGIES. Romaine and green lettuce, leafy greens, spinach, cucumber, carrot, zucchini, asparagus, broccoli, kale, onions, garlic, arugula, bok choy, dandelion greens, beets—the list goes on and on. You can chop these bad boys up in a bag for snacks or get organic frozen veggies to keep in the freezer. Organic smoothies are a great option for snacks. Non-starchy veggies are freebies—eat as many as you like! When possible, choose organic, seasonal, and local produce. In the winter months or when your favorite produce is out of season, you can find organic versions in the freezer section.

LOW GLYCEMIC FRUIT. Berries of all kinds, green apple, grapefruit, and nectarines are good choices.

CANNED FOODS. Fresh is best, but when not in season or if you're in a hurry, organic canned veggies and beans are minimally processed at the height of ripeness, often in the field, and make good bases for veggies stews and soups.

STOCK. Boxes of organic veggie, mushroom, fish, and chicken stock are ready starters for sauces, soups, and stews. I like to make my own stock, but if time and kitchen space is an issue, the best ready-made brands are healthy and acceptable.

HEALTHY OILS. Extra virgin coconut, grapeseed, cold-pressed extra virgin olive, flax, sesame, and avocado oils add great flavor to any dish you make.

RAW NUTS. Cashews (my fave), macadamias, almonds, hazelnuts, brazil nuts, and pecans add healthy fat and a bit of crunch to salads and side dishes. Plus, they are a great snack. Sprouted nuts are easier for digestion.

SEAWEED. It is a crispy snack (chip replacement) or can be a nice topper for salads and veg dishes.

SEEDS. Sesame, sunflower, hemp, chia, flax, and pumpkin seeds all add flavor and texture to salads, raw and cooked veggies, and other dishes.

NUT BUTTERS. Almond butter, cashew butter, walnut butter, and tahini (sesame seed paste) are preferable to peanut butter. Aside from triggering allergic reactions in some people, peanuts are actually a legume and so may be harder to digest than tree nuts. Use nut butters as spreads or thinned with a bit of water and used as a dressing on veggies, salads, and soba noodles.

> "I instantly feel the positive effects of eating well, just as I immediately feel the negative effects of eating poorly. Eating well and staying away from things that inflame my system are important. I don't eat meat, and I don't eat processed junk. I eat a lot of veggies, especially leafy greens, and I drink lots of water. It's really basic, healthy eating."
>
> Kaitlyn Lennon

SPICES. Turmeric, ginger, cinnamon, garlic, cayenne, clove, chili powder, cumin, paprika, pink Himalayan sea salt or gray sea salt, and fresh ground pepper are great go-to flavorings for all your savory dishes. These spices also have major healing properties and can help reduce inflammation in your body.

HERBS. Thyme, rosemary, parsley, basil, cilantro, and oregano are healthy and add flavor to so many dishes.

PROTEIN. Choose clean, lean sources of protein, such as wild-caught fish, free-range chicken, omega-3-enriched eggs, and grass-fed beef. No hormones or antibiotics used ever.

GLUTEN-FREE GRAINS. Quinoa, millet, amaranth, brown rice, 100 percent buckwheat, and soba noodles are all delicious alternatives to wheat-based pastas and wheat-based snacks.

BEVERAGES. Buy filtered or distilled water, or purchase a reverse-osmosis or Brita-filter pitcher to purify your water. Trust me, I have seen the pipes that the tap water runs through—*no bueno.* Purify all the way. Stock up on all kinds of teas so you can get creative with flavoring.

SWEETENER. Bye-bye aspartame; hello stevia.

CONDIMENTS AND ADD-ONS. Tahini (sesame seed paste); canned or jarred Kalamata olives; apple cider vinegar; balsamic vinegar; reduced-sodium, gluten-free tamari; reduced-sodium broth (vegetable or chicken); and Dijon mustard add layers of flavor to favorite dishes.

MILK SUBSTITUTES. Canned full-fat coconut milk and unsweetened hemp or almond milk are great substitutes for dairy milk.

SWEETS. About one ounce of dark chocolate per day is okay for a heart-healthy treat. Yum in the tum. Just make sure it's organic and at least 70 percent cocoa or higher. Avoid fillings like peanut butter, which could contain hydrogenated oils, and vanilla cream, which is just sugar and hydrogenated oil. Simple is best.

Cool Combo

How you eat is as important as what you eat. Especially for those of us in the CC Club, the goal is to have food move through our system effortlessly without putting loads of stress on it. Food combining can get pretty complicated, but for our purposes, let's start out with the basics.

Have you ever noticed after Thanksgiving dinner you feel inert and foggy-headed and the next day you still have a food hangover? I am sure you have had that sort of food coma after many meals. This coma mostly happens because you're mixing proteins with starch, and that's just not a good idea. News flash: we're supposed to feel sated and invigorated, not stuffed and exhausted, after finishing a meal. Did you know? I didn't. Now I do.

We're supposed to feel sated and invigorated, not stuffed and exhausted, after finishing a meal.

A strategy that I find useful in preventing after-dinner food paralysis and that I recommend to many of my clients is food combining. The idea behind food combining is to make things simpler for your body and your digestive system. When you simplify the components of a meal, your body can more efficiently, consistently, and easily process food and eliminate what's not needed.

Different forms of food move through your digestive system at different rates and speeds. A green juice or smoothie moves through your system much faster than brown rice or a piece of steak because the fiber in a juice or smoothie has been either removed or broken down, and your digestive system doesn't have to work as hard to access the nutrients and get rid of what's unnecessary. High-fiber or protein-dense foods, like brown rice and meat, give your digestive system a hard time; it takes longer for your system to break down grains and meat than it does to break down veggies.

So what happens when brown rice *and* a filet are forced to hang out together? Well, they can, and often do, cause a pile-up on the digestive highway. Honk, honk, get out of the way! The work required to break down and get nutrients from two kinds of heavy foods (starch, protein) contributes to your bloated, comatose, and ready-for-a-three-day-nap mood. Getting back to your Thanksgiving plate, it makes sense, right? Stuffing, turkey, mashed potatoes, gravy, with a few green

> "I have a 70/30 rule, which is to say 70 percent of the time I stick to small portions and simple meals. I avoid grains and wheat and focus on vegetables and easy-to-digest foods. I drink a lot of turmeric in hot water, as it's good for inflammation, or hot water with lemon. Then 30 percent of the time, I indulge in my favorite foods and treats. While I get so much joy and pleasure out of it, ultimately it gives me perspective and appreciation for my more simple day-to-day routine."
>
> Tara Sowlaty

beans on the side—turn on the radio, you're gonna be on that highway for a while. Not really great if you were planning on tossing around a football after dinner, or even just taking a walk or talking coherently to a friend.

If we know what foods to pair well together, everything will move through our digestive system more quickly, without leaving us feeling sluggish and stuffed. Food combining can get complicated. Here is a simple way to make it easy.

For instance, instead of having peanut butter on toast or a bagel and cream cheese to start your day, try a green smoothie. At lunch, instead of having a turkey sandwich with mayo, have a green salad with turkey. If you plan to have an animal protein like fish for dinner, pair it with steamed or sautéed spinach or another green veggie but lose the starch or grain. If you crave a baked sweet potato, lose the steak and pair it with veggies.

You see, you do not have to give up the protein and starch; you simply eat them at separate times. Make a choice to either have a starch meal (quinoa, sweet potato, millet, winter squash, etc.) with veggies or a protein meal (chicken, eggs, fresh fish, meat, etc.) with veggies. Try it out, see how you feel. By eating in a "light to heavy" way through the day, we give our body both the space to breathe and the tools it needs to help itself feel better.

FOOD COMBINING AND TRANSIT TIMES

Fruit
(15–30 MINUTES)
Eat Alone

Veggies
(2–3 HOURS)
Raw Veggies
Cooked Veggies
(low starch)

Starches
(2–3 HOURS)
Winter Squash
Sweet Potatoes
Grains (gluten free)
Avocado

Yes

Yes

Proteins
(4 HOURS)

Plant	Animal
Nuts	Chicken
Seeds	Fish
	Eggs

No
do not combine

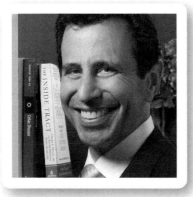

Gerard Mullin, MD

Gerard Mullin, MD, is an associate professor of medicine at the Johns Hopkins Hospital. He is board certified in internal medicine, gastroenterology, integrative medicine, functional medicine, and nutrition. Nationally and internationally renowned for his work in integrative gastroenterology and nutrition, Dr. Mullin has more than twenty years of clinical experience in the field of integrative gastroenterology and earned his master's degree in nutrition while in practice.

Here, Dr. Mullin talks about the importance of a healthy gut in terms of overall health and for managing chronic conditions.

From a medical perspective, a healthy gut contains a proper balance of friendly microbes and thoroughly digests and propels food through the digestive tract in a rhythmic fashion. The gut is the gateway to the body, as it serves as the interface of food, fomites (any object or substance capable of carrying infectious organisms, like germs and parasites), and foreign materials. If there is a hiccup in digestive function, the rest of the body is vulnerable to gut-derived bacterial toxins and environmental material. When your gut is not in good health, bacterial toxins can induce a systemic inflammatory response, which creates havoc on the body.

I always try to restore balance to the body through diet and lifestyle changes first before we try other interventions, including nutraceuticals, homeopathy, and naturopathy. The best way to promote gut health is through holistic living—a combination of diet and lifestyle. Foods that people should absolutely make staples in their diets include low-glycemic fruits (such as grapefruit, apples, and berries), vegetables, and probiotic, fermented foods. Wild-caught fish is another wonderful place to start when refocusing the ▶

▶ diet. Eat grains in moderation and red meat once in a while. Put your plate's focus on fiber-rich veggies, such as greens, including dandelion and kale. Eat a salad every day, dressed simply with olive oil and lemon juice. Keep it simple and whole.

The gut is not only sensitive to what you put in it. It's also very sensitive to your external environment and your perception of it. Eliminate or reduce the things that put you under stress. Avoid toxic relationships. Lack of sleep also affects the gut in negative ways. Get enough rest. Too many people depend on coffee and sugar to keep them going. A good diet, a low-stress external environment, and a solid night's sleep go a long way toward getting and keeping your gut in good shape. ■

Scrubbing Bubbles for Your Insides

Digestive enzymes are super important for your digestive system, as well as the rest of your body. You've probably heard of them, but what the heck are they?

We eat food, but our digestive system doesn't absorb *food*; it absorbs *nutrients*. Food has to be broken down into its nutrient pieces: amino acids (from proteins), fatty acids and cholesterol (from fats), and simple sugars (from carbohydrates), as well as vitamins, minerals, and a variety of other plant and animal compounds. Digestive enzymes are what do the breaking down. If we don't have enough of 'em, we can't break down our food, and our bodies can't absorb the nutrients. That means even if we are eating well, all that good stuff is not making its way into our body.

Disease in general can prevent proper digestive enzyme production. Celiac disease and Crohn's in particular can cause severe digestive enzyme problems. Even if you don't have a chronic issue directly related to digestion, your enzyme production could be in a funk, because chronic stress is a very common reason for digestive enzyme problems.

Promoting the effectiveness of your digestive enzymes can be done through your mouth. While a body in perfect balance doesn't need supplemental enzymes because it produces enough of them on its own, some of us might need some extra help. I take enzyme supplements with every meal; they come in a capsule and are widely available at health food and drug stores. There is also a lot we can do at the table to increase digestive enzymes. Luckily, eating to increase digestive enzymes fits right in with an alkaline-promoting diet and food combining. Don't you love it when that happens?

Here are my top tips for eating to support your enzymes:

Get raw. Digestive enzymes are most readily available when they come from raw foods, like fresh fruit and veggies.

Sprout out. Sprouted seeds and legumes have lots of digestive enzymes.

Ferment it. Add foods like sauerkraut, kimchee, and tempeh to your meals.

Go tropical. Papaya, pineapple, mango, and kiwi are significant sources of digestive enzymes.

Be Determined to Detox

Toxins are in your system. Believe it. Toxins represent the total amount of stressors on your system at any given time. Here are some of the things that contribute to our personal toxin load:

Take Time to Enjoy Your Food

Enjoying a meal is essential in eating well. Eat mindfully, slowly, and gently. Savor every morsel, and be happy when you eat. A peaceful, unhurried meal feeds your soul as much as the vitamins and minerals in what you are eating fuel your body.

▸ eating the SAD

▸ food allergies, environmental allergies, molds, and toxins from molds

▸ mental, emotional, and spiritual toxins

▸ some medications

▸ heavy metals, such as mercury and lead, petrochemicals, residues, pesticides, and fertilizers

▸ internal bacteria, fungus, and yeast

▸ hormonal and metabolic toxins

When our digestive system is overwhelmed with any one or more of these toxins, it gets overloaded. The key to my healing has been to detox every area of my life. The five most crucial ways to detox now:

DRINK PLENTY OF CLEAN WATER. Get at least eight to ten 8-ounce glasses of filtered water a day.

EXERCISE. This helps your blood and lymphatic system do their jobs.

BREAK A SWEAT. Try to break a sweat in some way every day. Even if that means sitting in the infrared sauna or steam room.

HEAL YOUR GUT. Ask your doctor about a gut-healing protocol.

DE-STRESS. De-stress and rid yourself of anger and anxiety through meditation, plenty of rest, spiritual practices, self-soothing techniques, and getting the mental and emotional support you need.

ELIMINATE PROPERLY. Keep your bowels moving, at least once or twice a day.

Taking out your internal trash is one of the most important things you can do for your body.

Taking Out the Trash: What Goes In Must Come Out

Keeping the body in a detox state or mode is essential to healing it. Pooping is a natural consequence of eating. If you put less stress on your system via food combining and eating an alkaline-supportive and fiber-rich diet, your body can focus on healing because your elimination system will be working properly and elimination will be less stressful for the body.

I know, I know—you are likely flinching just at reading the words "waste removal" or want to hide under the sheets at the words "bowel movement," but we are going to talk about it anyway, because taking out your internal trash is one of the most important things you can do for your body. You need to hear this. And let's face it: everybody poops. It's natural and one of the best things your body does, plus it's one of the first books you ever read.

Remember, our body is one machine with many moving parts working together, and the colon supports all parts of our being. This is what I know for sure. If we unclog the pipes and have a squeaky clean intestinal tract, and if we eat clean foods in combinations that support the digestive system and don't put pressure on it, we are definitely only helping our body rock. Our elimination system helps get rid of unnecessary waste from everything we have consumed and a bucket load of toxins that go with it.

Think about this: Did you know that a healthy body in tip-top shape should eliminate three to four times per day? Yes. You read that right: three to four times *a day.* Nourishing ourselves with the right foods is half the battle. We also need to make sure the unnecessary byproducts of the goodies we add into our diet have a clear passageway through which to effortlessly move straight to the dump (a.k.a. your throne, the toilet).

Okay, now that we have that covered and we broke the ice, *moving on!*

Good Chemistry

Paying attention to what goes in our body is always worthwhile, but sometimes a chronic health condition makes it tough to get *any* food into our bodies. Believe me, I know: I spent over a year unable to keep down any solid foods. Sometimes just adding the good stuff we talked about isn't enough. In times like these, we might need some extra help. I did.

For me, that extra help came from bio-chemical nutrition. Through blood analysis, supplementation, and nutrition, I was able to get back onto eating solid foods with no allergic reaction in one month alone.

If your chronic health conditions have severely compromised your digestive system and metabolism, or if you are doing everything "right" nutritionally but suspect it isn't enough, biochemical nutrition may be worth exploring.

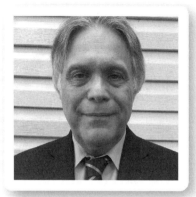

Terence Dulin,
DC, CTN, DCN, FAAIM

Terence Dulin is a chiropractor, certified naturopath, fellow in integrative medicine, and nutritionist in New York. He analyzes individuals' circumstances to identify and personalize specific diets and supplement programs for them.

Here, he gives an overview of biochemical nutrition, which deals with biochemical factors affecting our ability to maintain optimal health. ▶

When a person has a chronic illness or is on long-term medication due to a disease, the body changes its metabolism. The metabolism no longer works in the same mode as it does in someone who is healthy and not taking long-term medications. The more complex the illness, the harder it is for you to eat, absorb, process, and, finally, remove chemicals in your body. Biochemical nutritionists, like me, balance these factors by testing the blood and creating a diet and supplement program based on the results. If you have a chronic illness of any kind, it is worth having your blood tested for biochemical analysis. With the resulting information, a biochemical nutritionist can help your body chemistry achieve a balanced state and stop it from slowly sinking into new disease patterns.

Biochemical nutrition looks at an individual's body chemistry, lifestyle, stress, and environment to produce a program to keep the body as balanced and as functional as possible. While that program does not cure any disease, it does help keep the body running at optimum levels for a person's particular condition. Blood testing helps us keep track of progress and any changes in an individual's condition. Blood tests are snapshots of how an individual's body is functioning at a specific moment. Putting together many of them over time, we get an understanding of how the body works.

Once you have a chronic problem or are on medication long term, the rules for healthy lifestyles that apply to healthy people get thrown out the window. Everything you put into your body has negative and positive effects. An antibiotic may kill life-threatening bacteria, but can result in a negative effect, like a yeast infection. A medication that regulates your stomach acid may deplete your bone calcium and give you osteoporosis. What we do as biochemical nutritionists is work to minimize or remove these effects and keep our bodies balanced.

People with chronic conditions also need to consider how to avoid things that affect the way their medications work. You can no longer assume that because a food is considered "healthy" that it is good or safe for you. Fruit is healthy for most people, unless you have diabetes or a problem with metabolizing fructose. Then you should avoid fruit. Beef can be great to help get rid of anemia, but it will worsen gout and uric acid kidney stones. People with IBS (irritable bowel syndrome) do very poorly with raw vegetables; people with constipation may do great with them. Fish helps the immune system. But suppose you know your immune system is working too hard and attacking you, like it does when you have an autoimmune disease. By adding more foods that stimulate your immune system, you are, in fact, making yourself worse.

Understanding your own body's specific needs and problems is as important as knowing the functions on your cell phone. Medications are needed and are important weapons for your health, but meds are also very dangerous and need to be used as sparingly as possible. If you take care of your body chemistry properly through food and supplements, then you can either eliminate the need for medications or reduce them greatly.

When you embark on a program of biomedical nutrition, you have to start with a new paradigm: What fits in my biochemical factory for the least negative and most positive effect? The answer can be found in both food or diet and supplements. I mainly use vitamins, minerals, fatty acids, and amino acids to achieve results. These are natural body chemicals and tend to be very safe and effective. They are purified food without the calories, so to speak. We have to eat a lot more volume from food in order to get the nutrients we need to function.

Some nutrients, such as B-complex vitamins and vitamin C, are water soluble. Some, such as vitamins A, D, K, and E, are fat soluble and stay in your body. But we all have different absorption and use levels. The vitamin D3 levels are an example. Drinking a glass of milk fortified with vitamin D or playing in the sunshine was once considered to provide enough vitamin D for a person. Now rampant deficiencies have changed that view. So the supplements we use in biochemical nutrition are the ones your body knows how to use, because it does so on an everyday basis. They are very safe and effective.

In my practice I use vitamins, minerals, and amino acids more than other supplements. Most of the supplements I use are water soluble. We usually eat three times a day because water-soluble nutrients wash out of our body every four to six hours. Supplements, which are purified food for the most part, follow the same pattern, which is why I recommend taking them three times a day.

The U.S. Food and Drug Administration (FDA) regulates all supplement manufacturers that have Good Manufacturing Practice (GMP) certification for purity and strength. So look for brands with the GMP mark. ▪

▼ ▼ ▼

I hope you will refer to this chapter again and again as you shop, dine out, and prepare meals for yourself, your friends, and your family. Yes, do apply all this food information at home and do share your healthy meals with others! You can still enjoy eating and sharing a meal with friends and family while focusing on proper nourishment.

Just remember, it's less about removing all the things you currently love, and it's more about adding all of the good options you have that will help you. One step at a time. The most important thing I want you to remember about food is to make it whole, make it fresh, and make the time to truly enjoy its tastes and textures. You are what you eat, so cut the crap, and fuel and nourish your body accordingly. Bon appétit!

7

Movin' On Up

Until the time my body completely blew out at age twenty-five, I was a person who functioned in extremes. Go big or go home. Work hard; play harder. Work out six days a week, or don't do anything at all. This strategy worked for me—or so I thought. Chronic fatigue syndrome was the name of the game. My body was trying to get me to listen up and let it deeply rest. Instead of resting, I felt so weak and defeated that I physically (and spiritually) gave up. For months I just sat my ass on the couch watching reality TV and doing absolutely nothing to improve my physical state. Instead of trying to do as much as I could with ease, I did nothing, which didn't help anything at all whatsoever.

What I didn't know then was that my physical body needed *my attention and my presence*. When it was telling me to take a rest, it meant to do that with the intention of healing. My body was asking for my attention and my willingness to listen to it. When I was sick and searching for answers, I didn't understand that, so I allowed myself to feel depressed. I believed that my body just couldn't and wouldn't physically keep up with me anymore. Instead of loving it, I disconnected from it completely.

When I finally did drag my butt off the couch, I happened to see my reflection as I was passing by a mirror. I took a good hard look at myself. I was so swollen from idiopathic edema that I didn't even recognize myself. *Who is that?* I looked and felt like a foreigner in my skin. *No mas.* I was sick and tired of looking and feeling sick and tired. Feeling out of shape and not knowing where to turn, I broke out my dusty yoga mat and simply lay down in savasana (corpse pose). I let myself breathe there for ten minutes. Simply lying still with attention and connecting to my body through breath allowed me to get familiar with my body again, and I felt better. A light bulb went off. Through gentle movement and breath, I could support my body, reconnect with it, and help it to move better, despite my fatigue. Yoga and all of its healing benefits seemed to be calling my name.

One of my doctors had recommended restorative yoga as a way for me to calm my nervous system, relax, and get connected to my breath again. So I took my not-so-dusty old yoga mat, strapped it to my back, and went to see an older yogi who happened to be in a "temporary space," which when I showed up was not a yoga room—it was a tiny cubicle in the middle of Manhattan. In the next office, two lawyers threw tantrums and yelled at each other at the top of their lungs. Very Zen! *Ommmmmmm.* But at that point, I didn't care.

I just wanted someone to give me time and attention so I could figure out how to give those things to myself. In other words, I was desperate and seeking a way out of suffering.

The yogi propped me up on a bolster pillow and I sort of slumped over it. All I remember of what happened next is her nudging me and saying, "Amy, you can gently open your eyes." I woke up confused but *so* incredibly relaxed. I was with a complete stranger on the floor of an office cubicle, with the continued screaming and yelling of lawyers in the background, and I had just taken the nap of a lifetime. I hadn't felt that at peace in my body in years. It was then I realized the amazing benefits of restorative yoga. Even though I actually hadn't done much of it at that session, I was reminded that I had the ability to move, and that is a beautiful gift that some people don't have. I could still hear the lawyers' voices echoing in the hallway as I packed up my mat and went home.

After that, I started to do whatever I could to move and get back in touch with my physical strength and stamina. You too may not have the energy for much, but you can do *something.* Simply lying in a restorative yoga pose can help your nervous system calm down, your body relax, and your mind become still. Restorative yoga was my main source of movement for a long time, and boy, did it help me give my body the attention that it so deeply needed.

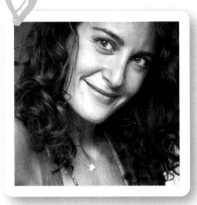

Elena Brower

My favorite yoga teacher, Elena Brower, talks about the great relief that restorative yoga can bring. Here, she explains how restorative yoga can be helpful for those of us with chronic conditions and offers five restorative yoga poses to try.

Restorative yoga is still and slow—as much about stilling your mind as it is about quieting your body, so your entire being can enter into a more nurturing, healing space. During restorative yoga poses, you focus on the rhythm of your breathing to invite your physical and mental bodies into alignment. Props like a block and a blanket may be used to help you hold the poses for a longer time. The longer you hold a restorative yoga pose, the greater the benefit.

When you feel tired after a workout, a restorative yoga session can profoundly refresh you. Those with chronic issues may begin using this or any yoga practice with care and patience.

These restorative poses will help lend space to your mind and your body. Even a simple pose like placing your legs up a wall helps you look at your life from a new perspective. It helps you come back to your natural, healing state. Notice how each of these postures helps you feel more expansive and present.

Urdhva Baddha Hastasana/ Upward Bound Hand Pose

Stand at the front of your yoga mat, palms facing forward, hands at your sides, feet touching. Lift the sides of your waist and the back of your heart away from the floor as you inhale and reach your arms up to the sky, turning your interlaced palms to face the ceiling. ▶

Stretch long and tall with your next inhalation and then exhale. Feel into your body as you take this momentary snapshot of your inner being. Notice any spaces in your body that feel closed, and send your breathing—the light of your attention—there.

Release your hands back down to your sides and close your eyes for a moment. Feel the resonance of that stretch in your shoulders and upper arms and heart. Take a moment to see how you feel now.

After a couple of breaths, interlace your hands, switching to the non-habitual interlacing, and bring your hands up overhead to turn them inside out, palms facing the ceiling. Root your feet down into the floor and breathe deeply. This should feel very stabilizing.

Lower your arms, rest your hands at your sides, and close your eyes. It takes only seconds for these movements to bring us into our heart, where we can feel more resonance and connection to ourselves. Once again, take a snapshot of your interior space, how you feel inside.

Baddha Konasana/Bound Angle

Begin seated on your mat. Place a bolster, folded blankets, couch cushion, or two firm pillows directly beneath the back of your seat. Bring the soles of your feet to touch. Press your feet into one another, widen your seat back behind you, and slowly fold down.

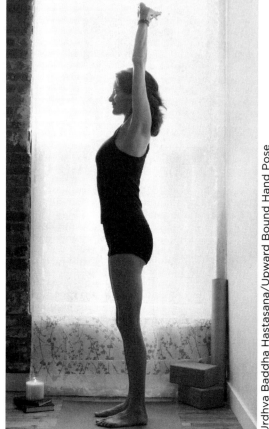

Urdhva Baddha Hastasana/Upward Bound Hand Pose

Be clear with yourself and breathe directly into your boundary here, without trying to change anything. When we start to try to fix things—a very human and habitual choice—we lose contact with reality. Whatever it is that you are managing today, see it, observe it—all of its facets, aspects, weirdness, and wonderfulness. The moment you see it without trying to fix it, you're moving toward a more healing inner state. And in that moment, there is a solution lingering in your observation.

Slowly inhale as bring your torso back up.

through the lens of blame, your work is to stand in front of that perspective and choose another possible view; that is your responsibility and privilege.

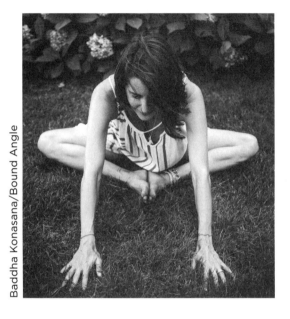

Baddha Konasana/Bound Angle

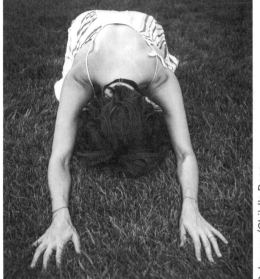

Balasana/Child's Pose

Balasana/Child's Pose

Sit on the floor on your knees, with your knees together. Fold your torso forward toward the floor. Let your arms extend and rest in front of you; turn your gaze to the right or let your forehead rest on the floor.

Take this time to bow to those you've been blaming. Bow with gratitude and devotion; they've given you a map to your highest way of seeing. If you've been seeing them

Viparita Karani/Legs Up the Wall

Set your bolster up against the wall, with the long edge against the wall. Scoot your tush up onto the bolster, and move your sitting bones as close as possible to the wall. Lengthen your legs up the wall with your seat and sacrum on the bolster; rest your head and shoulders on the floor. With your legs up the wall, relax your body and hold space for yourself. ▶

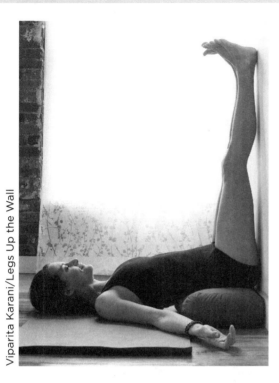

conditions of opening, softening every system in your body (nervous, lymphatic, circulatory, respiratory, digestive). Relax your hands and all the muscles of your face. Notice the weight of your hands on the floor.

To come off the wall, gently bend your knees and place the soles of your feet on the wall. Press away from the wall so you can comfortably roll to your right and rest there in fetal position for a moment. Roll off the bolster and onto the floor.

Savasana/Corpse Pose

Return to your mat and arrange a bolster, two blankets, pillows, towels, or a couch cushion so they will be beneath your middle back when you lie down. This support should extend down to your mid thighs. Position a block or books to prop up your feet. Rest your ankles on another bolster or rolled blanket.

Be completely passive and yet awake. Take a full look at how you feel. Your entire being, quiet, healing, receptive, listening. ■

▸ This is a very relaxing posture, especially if you spend a lot of time on your feet or in a seat. Let your arms rest at your sides and invite nourishing circulation from your feet into your organs. You are creating the

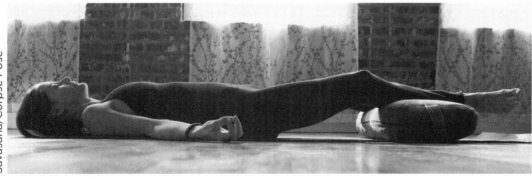

Easy Does It

If it's been a while since you've done consistent and sustained exercise, ease into it, by engaging in your favorite activity one day and then taking the next one off. Repeat that pattern to build up your strength and to condition your body for the next step.

When I was living back at my childhood home in Philadelphia and regaining my strength, I made a pact with myself that I would walk as far as I could five days a week, even if I ended up making it just a block or two. I held myself accountable to that, and eventually I was walking impressive distances on a daily basis. At that point I was able to add in more vigorous forms of movement.

You can start with a short-term goal that you can stick to and accomplish, just as I did. For instance, commit to taking a ten-minute walk five days a week. Consider getting a pedometer to count your steps and try increasing steps by two hundred to four hundred each time you take a walk. Or how about going from ten minutes every day you walk to twenty minutes?

You always have to understand your current limits before you can stretch them—and stretch them you should. You'll get stronger, fitter, and happier if you do. If walking is your thing, you can add in some light wrist or hand weights to get in a bit of upper body resistance training. A 2½- to 5-pound weight in each hand will add to the challenge of your

> "Lying on my yoga mat and doing simple stretches and gentle twists gives me a mental power shift, and it gets the lymphatic system going. Dancing and grooving to music always gives me a mood boost as well; it's really one of my favorite things to do!"
>
> *Tara Sowlaty*

walk. But again, set yourself new goals only when you're ready.

Do what works best for you and what you like to do: jumping rope, swimming, strength training, running, hula hooping, dancing, rebounding, four- or seven-minute intense workouts, or high-energy low-impact aerobics. Once your chosen exercise has become a habit (twenty-one days of it, and you'll be there), ramp up your goals. Embrace your inner Jane Fonda. If you need some more motivation, get yourself a pink velour tracksuit or some leg warmers and get out there and work those legs!

You too may not have the energy for much, but you can do something.

"When you find workouts that you actually enjoy, you literally look forward to getting the time to do it. For me it's all about either getting pumped by the music or connecting to nature. When I'm not feeling up to it, I check in and remind myself that I always feel so happy afterward. Moving my body, disconnecting from the world around me, leaving my phone behind, and just being with myself in a focused way feels amazing!

What works for me is to schedule my workouts into my week, just like any other meeting so they become a natural part of my week. And I remind myself that I am extremely grateful to even have the chance to get up and move. Others don't have that option because of their illnesses or what have you, and I never ever want to take that for granted."

Tara Sowlaty

Pedal to the Metal

As I started to feel better, I wanted to add more cardio to my fitness routine. It was time for some boot camp, one made specifically for me. I had so many health issues bogging me down that I didn't even know where to start. So I started journaling about what brought me joy as a child, and I remembered how much

I loved jumping on a trampoline. Luckily, rebounders or mini trampolines were in, so it was easy to find one I could use at home, and it was easy to find rebounder classes near my house. I pushed myself slowly by doing low-impact exercises, and I started to breathe again in a different way. My body rewarded me with so many benefits, but the best one was feeling stronger and stronger with each effort I made. That strength was *mine.* I owned it, and I felt powerful after years of feeling like I was sitting side by side next to myself.

Every time I doubted my strength, I would say to myself, "I am a warrior. My strength is unlimited." I would repeat it in my head as a mantra: "I am a warrior. My strength is unlimited." As I jumped on the trampoline and my legs ached, I would say to myself, "I am a warrior. My strength is unlimited." I repeated this phrase until I believed it and knew it to be true. My thought became my reality. I felt very fatigued, but I wanted to prove myself wrong about not being able to build up my stamina and ability to exercise for a sustained period; when I accomplished one physical activity, I wanted to show I could do another, more difficult, activity.

I took my out-of-shape butt (no self hate, just honesty) to a fitness and movement studio for a fitness evaluation. My trainer kicked that soft, not-so-cute butt into gear. It was challenging. I was completely deconditioned. There were times where it felt so hard I

Get moving in any way you can, as much as you can, as often as you can.

wanted to curl into a ball and give up or just cry because I felt so sad and like I couldn't go any farther. I didn't quit because I believed there was more inside of me than I was telling myself. My trainer kept reminding me of that when I seemed to have lost my momentum.

As I saw my physical ability improving, I started to feel stronger emotionally and spiritually, as well as physically. I felt free. The Glow Warrior spirit was born here. In fact, it was right in the middle of Katy Perry's "Part of Me" when the chains of inactivity, pain, and self doubt broke and fell off to the floor. I proved myself wrong; I could exercise and move—and enjoy it. Exercise has now become a ritual that connects me to that Glow Warrior spirit. I went from a full-blown, totally deconditioned, two-year couch potato to a strong, willful, connected *survivor*. Exercise and movement made me feel as if I were capable of anything I set my mind to.

All you have to do is choose to believe that you can do more than you think you can. Get moving in any way you can, as much as you can, as often as you can. Movement is

a privilege we have that we need to treasure, honor, and use! Our amazing bodies were made to move. Even when you feel achy, tired, stiff, you name it, simple stretches make your body feel so much better.

Easy tiger! I am not telling you to get off the couch, do eighty pushups, twenty sets of high knees, and go run a half marathon. Your body is going through a lot and needs some extra tender lovin' care. Yet in order to heal, your body also needs to move in some way so that your blood is circulating; one small thing every day is good start. This can simply be taking a walk for as long as you can. It could mean taking a work-out class if you feel up to it, or putting on your favorite feel-good song and dancing to it. It could mean taking a gentle restorative yoga class. Just move—whatever movement your body can do. Honor your body.

There are plenty of days when I'd rather stay in bed or just skip the workout and

Simple acts of movement can boost your happiness levels, and the way your body feels, in just a few minutes.

Exercise: You Can't Beat the Benefits

Exercising doesn't just help your figure go from a zero to a ten on the hotness scale. Lot's of irresistibly great things happen when you make movement a regular part of your weekly routine:

- better sex
- smoother, younger skin
- deeper, more restful sleep
- bigger brain power (yup, exercise makes you smarter)
- improved digestion
- more robust immune system
- stronger bones
- lower blood pressure
- healthier cholesterol levels
- energized endorphins (movement is a real mood lifter)

head straight for the couch, computer, or the office. But I drag myself up to do something even when I feel like a big bowl of crappiness because when I lie around and do nothing, that laziness feeds on itself. If you lie about all day, your blood gets stagnant, making you feel worse. That's because being active boosts high-density lipoprotein (HDL), the

so-called good cholesterol, and decreases unhealthy triglycerides. This keep your blood flowing smoothly, which decreases your risk of cardiovascular diseases.

I force myself to do something physical every day. If it's nice out, I'll go rollerblading in the park. If it's raining, I'll take a class or do resistance work with a motivating trainer. If nothing happens to appeal to me on a particular day, I'll take a long walk with my favorite empowering playlist on my iPod and get my strut on. I recently learned boxing, and I absolutely *love* it. Not only is it an awesome full-body workout, but it is also very helpful for releasing any pent-up anger or resentment—at myself, my docs, my friends, the world, whatever. Pow! Zap! Jab, cross jab! Gone! And no one gets hurt. You totally deserve a Rocky moment—give it a shot. Kick ass and take names!

What did you do as a kid that made you feel free? What did you love to do that was fun? Start there. For me it was rebounding; for you it could be hula hooping or jumping rope, or just putting on your favorite song and letting loose. Whatever it was, reconnect with what brought you joy.

The bottom line: you're never going to stick with a fitness and movement program if you don't enjoy doing it. Have you ever really thought about things you like to do? Well, let's do it right now. We'll come back to your answers later in the chapter.

- What activities bring you joy?

- Which ones can you start doing today?

- How many minutes can you exercise today, right now?

- Are there activities you never tried but would like to try (e.g., spinning, paddle boarding, the tango)?

- When can you exercise (at night, in the morning)?

Pick an exercise that makes you feel free or reminds you what joy and freedom feel like in your body. Then pick a mantra that empowers you and say it while you are doing the exercise. Can't think of one? Use mine! "I am a warrior. My strength is unlimited." Make it yours.

Any movement (even if it's small) always makes you feel so much better. So get shaking on your way to becoming a Glow Warrior! Commit to something. Your butt, abs, arms, *and mood* will thank you later for it.

Get Your Tush on the Happy Train

Illness, especially a chronic health issue, can make you feel as if your body has abandoned you. Put the hate that you feel for your body behind you, and learn to love it again with easy, gentle movement and, when you are ready, sweat-inducing exercise that uplifts your mood and honors your physical abilities. Your body is your temple. It is the house in which you live. It is your job to honor it. Getting fit and staying fit is a state of mind. Just because you feel like a big blob on some days (and you know which days I'm talking about) doesn't mean that feeling has to be your vibe all day, every day. Simple acts of movement can boost your happiness levels, and the way your body feels, in just a few minutes.

The increased blood flow movement brings also benefits your noggin almost immediately. That's why you often feel clear and focused after a workout, a long walk, or a hike. Exercising regularly supports the growth of new brain cells, and we can all use a few more of those. One of the most effective and noninvasive ways to fight depression (so common among members of the Chronic Condition Club) is exercise.

Mark Hyman, MD, says:

Exercise is essential for good health. It is the best antidepressant and anti-anxiety medication available. It reduces inflammation, improves mood, balances neurotransmitter function, and increases neuroplasticity and neurogenesis, just to mention a few of the positive effects it has on your brain. If exercise could be put in a pill, it would be the biggest blockbuster medication of all time. Unfortunately, today, nearly half of Americans live a sedentary lifestyle and 88 percent don't get enough exercise. No wonder we have an epidemic of broken brains![1]

A recent study at the University of Alabama at Birmingham shows that exercise boosts the mood of people managing chronic conditions, not to mention the mood of everyone else on the planet.[2] And there's more: Alan J. Gelenberg, MD, chair of the Department of Psychiatry at Penn State University, says the study's findings are consistent with the American Psychiatric Association, which recommends regular exercise to help combat the blues often associated with those dealing with chronic conditions.[3] The study showed that even moderate exercise makes a difference.

You can do this: just thirty minutes a day for five days is what you should be going for. It's not a huge amount of time; there are twenty-four hours in a day, and we're just asking for thirty minutes a day! Consistency is key. Keep up the good work, and the good work will reward you with a good mood and a great ass.

"I have an app on my phone that helps me get close to ten thousand steps a day. I also love to do squats holding my daughter or throwing her up in the air because she giggles every time.

When my MS acts up, I tend to jog and run more because I want to always be sure that I can. It is a disconcerting feeling to think your ability to walk or jog could be compromised, and making sure it isn't is important to me, emotionally and physically."

Lindsay White

Science Lesson:
Your Body on Exercise

There's so much good news about moving your booty and twirling your tummy. Exercise, especially consistent vigorous movement, helps normalize glucose, insulin, and leptin levels. (Leptin is the "satiety hormone" that inhibits hunger.) This normalization is a crucial factor in preventing many lifestyle-related chronic diseases, like hypertension and type-2 diabetes.

A lot of other great things happen in your body when you exercise. Your heart pumps more blood and much-needed oxygen to your hard-working muscles. Oxygen is the gas your muscles need to run. If your car runs out of gas, you're stranded. Likewise, when the muscles don't get enough oxygen, you're stranded—on your couch.

Not only that, but every intricate element of your system gets a boost when you exercise. Your heart gets stronger, and its left ventricle gets larger, which is awesome because the left ventricle increases the heart's capacity for pumping out larger volumes of oxygen-saturated blood per beat. Put that in the win column! It's the difference between a full gas tank in a Ferrari and a low tank in a Rent-a-Wreck.

A network of capillaries brings that oxygen-rich blood to every single muscle fiber in your body, and when you exercise, they multiply. Woo-hoo! It's like earning interest at the bank. More good news: your muscles get better at accessing the oxygen they need. When every muscle fiber has more capillaries surrounding it, like an adoring crowd of fans, the supply of nutrients and oxygen to muscle fibers increases. Can you feel the love?

Fresh Air, Fresh Mind

Whether you end up doing digital Zumba and yoga classes in your living room or joining a gym to sweat with your friends, you still have to get outside every day. A lot of us are suffering from nature deficit disorder, which is not yet an actual medical diagnosis, but it's the idea, put forth by journalist Richard Louv, to describe the terrible impact losing our

> "I had to mourn the death of my running, and it was upsetting to me at first. But once I embraced that my body wanted a change, I found Pilates. While it doesn't give me that high running gave me, it's something new, and I really like it. It's a lot of core work, and I can get a good workout with no pressure on my feet and no pain."
>
> Morgan Segal

connection to nature has on our well-being.[4] In fact, research shows that exercising outside has more benefits, both physical and psychological, than doing the same exercise inside. I try to make it a point to take long walks outside and get away from the city as often as possible. I love hiking, doing yoga outside, or just simply sitting and taking in the fresh air with the sun on my face, which is very restorative and healing for me.

A study from the Peninsula College of Medicine and Dentistry found that data from numerous exercise studies showed that exercising in natural environments was associated with greater feelings of revitalization, increased energy, decreased tension and depression, and greater enjoyment and satisfaction with outdoor activities than indoor activities. The test

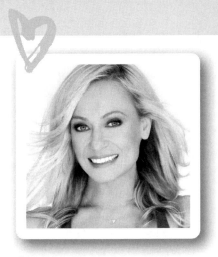

Simone De La Rue

Simone De La Rue began training in classical ballet at the age of three and enjoyed a successful dance career that spanned more than two decades, including numerous performances on Broadway in New York City, London's West End, and her native Australia. Simone has always had a passion for fitness and health. As a dancer, she studied yoga and Pilates, and she developed Body By Simone (BBS) using the techniques she used to train and practice as a dancer. Body By Simone mixes dance with yoga and Pilates to develop your core strength, create long lean muscle, and improve your cardio fitness, so you can reach the ultimate goal of having a dancer's body.

Simone shares her thoughts on exercising when you're a member of the Chronic Condition Club and why rebounding, in particular, can be helpful.

My attitude toward exercise, especially for those with chronic health issues, is let's see what happens and experiment to find out what kind of movement will work for you and your body. Of course, I love rebounding on the trampoline because it's so good for lymphatic glands and draining fluids. The low impact of the trampoline is brilliant for getting the heart rate up. But it is still low-impact cardio, so it's a great place to start for someone who hasn't moved in awhile. I call it jumping for joy because it's also so good for the soul and the spirit.

If you can't find a rebound class or you just want to invest in a home rebounder, get the best one you can afford. I use JumpSport; they can be used at home, they are lightweight, and the mat is very good quality. You can rebound every day since it's a low-impact activity, and it won't hurt your joints or tire the muscles.

I recommend purchasing a heart-rate monitor and finding a safe place to work out. Get yourself some resistance bands; they can travel with you, and they give you a lot of control over how hard you work. They work the muscles without overloading them, helping you build long, lean muscles most women want. We do high reps with the bands and with hand weights as well—low weight (two to four pounds) and high reps. ■

subjects also said they were much more likely to repeat the outdoor activity.[5]

Doing something outside is often more fun than doing it at the stinky old gym or the confines of your bedroom. How much more interesting is it to take a long walk in the woods or even on the sidewalk, for example, than it is to walk on a treadmill? Think of how much more fun your yoga session would be at the beach or in the backyard than inside a not-so-Zen fluorescent-lit room. Get outside, say hello to the leaves and grass, kiss a cow (not on the lips!), and commune with Mother Nature. She loves you!

Make Friends with Your Lymph System

The lymph system, a major part of the body's immune system, carries nutrients to cells and then bathes every cell with them. It also washes away waste products from your cells. Think of the lymphatic system as the metabolic waste disposal system of the body. It rids the body of toxins, such as dead and cancerous cells, nitrogenous wastes, infectious viruses, heavy metals, and other assorted junk the cells don't want or need.

Unlike your arterial system, the lymphatic system does not have its own pump. Instead, the lymph system doesn't move unless *you* move; it is completely dependent on physical exercise. Without movement, cells are left to stew in their own waste products; meanwhile, they are crying out for nutrients. This double trouble can lead to arthritis, cancer, and other degenerative diseases.

Rebounding or bouncing on a large exercise ball provides the movement necessary to help your lymphatic system to do its job and drain those killjoys away. So do jumping jacks, jump rope, dance, and run. Yoga and Pilates, two of my other favorite exercises, also help stimulate the lymph system, as well as help with overall core strength and fitness levels. I especially love rebounding, however, because there is something about the rhythm of hopping on a trampoline that frees you from the prison of pain that chronic conditions often put you in, making you feel like a free, fun-loving kid again. In short, it's a blast.

Muscle In on Some Action

Building muscle is important for strength, fat burning, and overall tone and leanness. We all need to be strong, but there's no need to compete with the muscle heads for a spot on a sweaty weight machines. Mat Pilates and resistance bands offer two ways to build that muscular strength, right at home.

Mat Pilates is a gentle, low-impact, but serious strength-training exercise. It is a precise method of movement and stretching that strengthens your core, abdomen, and pelvis, and doing Pilates improves your mood almost immediately. It's also amazing for optimizing your posture and increasing flexibility. The good news is all you need is a mat and an at-home instructional video.

Resistance bands allow you to do an effective strength-training routine without the need for a set of bulky, heavy weights. With just three or four different-sized bands, you can get a full body workout with lots of variety and various levels of challenge. Best of all, resistance bands are inexpensive, stow away easily, and can even travel with you, so there's never an excuse not to work those muscles—even when you're on the road.

Chart Your Fitness Course

The best way to keep track of your fitness goals and accomplishments is to track them. There are loads of resources to help you do this, especially online. But sometimes having something tangible right in front of you is a bit more motivating than logging into a website, which can be, frankly, easier to ignore. Find a pretty journal, put your name on it, and start writing down what you're doing every day to move to your body and take note of how you feel about it. Remember, love, whatever you think you can't do, you *can* do more, for five minutes more.

▼ ▼ ▼

Now you have all of the tools and information you need to get moving and grooving. You can do it! The ability to move is a blessing, and by choosing to move, you are showing respect for that great privilege. You are rooting for yourself and your body, and you are giving your body the attention it deserves. Your mind makes the choice before your body to succeed with movement. Choose to drop the chronic condition chains that keep you thinking you can't exercise. Let them go—there is no better time than now.

8

Find Your Spiritual Center

Connecting with my soul has been one of the best things I have ever done for my physical condition and my mind. Finding my soul was like finding my home, and when I found it, everything else started to flow, and my body started to heal.

Even though I was raised Jewish, I don't consider myself a particularly religious person in the traditional or orthodox sense. When my bat mitzvah came along, I was more excited about the 60s theme of my party and how rad the Janis Joplin centerpiece was than I was about the actual ritual. But I am very connected to the Jewish culture, especially the emphasis it places on the family and community, and its other tribal aspects.

Making my early religious experience even more eclectic, I went to Quaker school growing up. It played a very big and important role in my appreciation for spiritual matters. Each Wednesday, the school set aside an hour for group reflection, called Meeting for Worship. The Quakers have a very strong sense of community and unity, and this group practice spoke to me. I

looked forward to it. It was a special time of day when we could stop and think quietly or collectively. Some (many) students dreaded Wednesdays, but I absolutely loved Meeting for Worship because it was one of the very few times that I had to sit still and just *be*, where I could be silent and reflect in a community of other people who were doing the same thing. I had never experienced silence and reflection in this way before, and it became my favorite part of the whole school week. Without having this time scheduled for me, it would have been easy to forget along the way, especially because I was in middle and high school and easily distracted. At the time I had no idea how crucial silent reflection is to our ability to truly thrive, and after I left Quaker school, I didn't make time for it. Now I know how important self-reflection is, and I have learned to schedule the time in for myself before anything else.

The debilitating physical pain I had as a young teenager disrupted the development of my internal compass. When my illness was at its peak later in my life, I delved more deeply into spirituality. Dealing with illness and trying to heal myself at times felt like walking the plank all by myself. I was totally desperate, seeking a way out of my suffering. There were moments where I felt so isolated and so alone. I felt that not a soul in the world understood how I felt. What I realized through seeking is that the person who was inside of me before I got sick was *still* inside of me; I just was having trouble hearing her.

The pain took me on a detour away from peace and into fear. So I assure you that the person inside yourself is still there, exactly as she was before the whole mess of chronic illness started. She is whole. She is your essence. She is your spirit. All you have to do to get back in touch with her is believe that things will change. Believe that there is a better life for you than the one you have now. Believe that no matter what the diagnosis, there is a better, more positive reality waiting for you when you open the door for it. When you commit to believing, everything shifts, and you make room for that being inside and for a better version of life.

I have always been a seeker of connecting to something greater than me; I just never had the resources to find what I was looking for. When I was first sick, I started to read a lot of unfamiliar books by people who are now my greatest teachers and mentors. A lot of them are experts featured in this book. They all talked about the connection to self and quality of life. At first, I didn't know what they were talking about exactly, but it sounded appealing and real, and I knew that I wanted it for myself. At the darkest time in my life, when I felt utterly hopeless, Kris Carr's book *Crazy Sexy Cancer Survivor* fell into my lap. I read it straight through while I was tucked away in my childhood bed. I devoured it. I had been unable to focus or read for well over a year (or so I told myself that), and my inner guide found this book, put it in my lap, and I didn't look up until the final page. That is when my light bulb went off and everything shifted for me. Here was this woman who chose to have a quality of life much greater than her diagnosis was ever going to hand to her. I sought out meditation. I went to a lot of yoga classes, and then I sat in on some really intriguing courses on dharma and Buddhism, as well as classes about approaching life in a mindful way. The teachers all spoke similarly about how life itself is much less important than how we relate to life. Whoa. I heard that, and *that* was that for me.

I have taken the spiritual part of each of the religions I have been around and incorporated them into my spiritual practice. It's so important for people in the CC Club to find a way to connect with the divine, the universe, God, or whatever it is for you. Don't worry about names and labels; all you have to know is that your spirit, your soul, is the nonphysical part of you that is the seat of your emotions and character. When something deeply painful happens to us in our lives, knocking the wind out of us and rocking us to our core, like chronic conditions can and do, we need something to believe in. If we don't have a belief in something hopeful, we remain hopeless. If we don't believe that we will get better, we will never get better. We must find faith.

If spiritual practices are new to you, don't get bogged down by the details. When the spirit moves you, let it groove you! A spiritual center gives you sustenance, a place to go when things look bleak *and* when things are great because it's a balancing place, where you can be present with your feelings without judgment or harshness. In your center is stillness. In your center is peace. We have to embark on the journey to our heart center in order to access, embrace, and reconnect with our spirit. This spiritual center is available inside of you 24/7, and as you deepen your spiritual practice, you will be able to connect with it at a moment's notice.

Chronic illness can be very isolating. Finding a spiritual center brings you balance, peace, and introspection, as well as softness and compassion. While your spiritual center is extremely personal, it also draws you closer to like-minded people—exactly the kind of people you need in your life in order for you to thrive and blossom.

The Spirit Calls

Set up your smartphone to send you a daily (or more frequent) reminder to pause for ninety seconds, close your eyes, and just breathe and be with yourself. It's so easy to forget or put off connecting with our spirit during busy days. While going on a retreat or staying at an ashram is plenty spiritual, the times we really need sustenance for our soul is when we are in the thick of our lives. If technology can help you find moments to reflect and be grateful, by all means use it.

Take a Deep Breath

There is a place deep within each and every one of us that contains overwhelming love, serenity, and peace. When we are struggling in our physical body and worrying about a million things that *could* go wrong or that *might* happen or that "will be," we are completely disconnected from our heart center, where love lies, and we are living in a place of constant fear. In other words, when we're not living in the present; we're stuck in an unknown and unknowable future that is controlled and rooted in fear. The opposite of fear is love. The more we can focus on the present, the more we can feel and receive love.

The best way to start to access our heart center and bring ourselves back to the present moment is through conscious breathing. While I was trying to "get better" and deal with my newfound, not-so-fun reality, it was as though I was holding my breath. When I embraced meditation and deep breathing, they were a revelation.

Proper breathing has a positive, noticeable effect on our health. The following three-part breath exercise is one of the most powerful breathing techniques you can do, and it can be done anywhere at anytime. Here's how it's done:

1 Sitting comfortably, close your eyes, and take a deep breath into your abdomen through your nose, so your tummy expands like a balloon.

2 Continue inhaling to expand your ribcage with air.

3 Continue inhaling to further expand the breath into your chest.

4 Reverse the sequence by exhaling out through your mouth first from the chest, then from the ribcage, and then from the abdomen.

5 Once you have exhaled all the air, repeat the three-part inhale and three-part exhale

as many times as you need to bring yourself back to a calm and present center.

Here's another breathing technique that I have used. It calms the nervous system and brings us back from any fight-or-flight feelings that might be coursing through us.

1 Sit still and tall. Close your eyes and breathe through your nose.

2 Inhale for a count of two. Hold the breath in for a count of one. Exhale gently, counting to four. Keep your breathing even and smooth.

3 Breathe this way for at least five minutes to see a genuine change in your mood.

Miss Diagnosis: Shifting Your Beliefs

When we are diagnosed with something, we mentally, physically, and spiritually hear that diagnosis as a limitation, something permanent that we need to adjust to, a wound that will never heal, if you will. If we believe that limitation is our reality forever and ever, our spirit will break or be injured or bruised. That is where faith and belief come in.

For example, when I heard a doctor say that my colon would never work again, I believed him. I truly believed that I would never find a cure and my only way out was surgery. After I had established a true spiritual practice (at the time of that pronouncement, I had none), I knew and believed that my colon would work again. This simple shift in belief got my ass to many more specialists, who had much more information and knowledge than the original doctor, and who had bucket loads of more solutions and suggestions, as well as a medication that worked specifically on my exact motility issue. When my thyroid doctor said that my thyroid was under so much stress it had essentially shut itself off, I believed that my thyroid would never work again. Wrong. Now I believe that my medicine will work and create harmony and balance for me exactly as it should.

What beliefs about your diagnosis are you willing to shift? Think of a diagnosis you've been given. For instance, maybe you've been told, "Your fibromyalgia will keep you in constant pain and feeling exhausted." Write down that diagnosis.

Now, think about what a contrary belief would be. For the fibromyalgia example, how about, "I am pain free and energetic."

A couple other examples:

DIAGNOSIS "Your arthritis may incapacitate you."

BELIEF "I am completely healthy and well. My body works and moves freely just as it is supposed to."

DIAGNOSIS "You will not be able to walk."

BELIEF "I will dance."

Write down your chosen contrary belief and sit with it for a while. Hear it in your mind. Does it feel delicious? Does the thought make you happy? Does it resonate through every cell in your body? Is it your dream? I want the idea of it to give you chills. If it doesn't, it needs to be rewritten. When the reality of your chosen belief sounds like something you yearn for, something that would make you your happiest you, you have your mantra. You can add this mantra to your deep breathing practice.

> "I do have my faith, but I am not a religious person. My spiritual practice is taking a bath every night. It's that simple. Taking twenty minutes every night for myself to be alone with my thoughts and just relax helps me keep mentally clear and able to give of myself to my family, work, and friends."
>
> *Lindsay White*

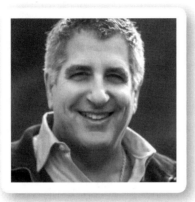

Joel M. Evans, MD

Joel M. Evans, MD, a board certified obstetrician/gynecologist and international lecturer, is the founder and director of the Center for Women's Health in Stamford, Connecticut, where he practices integrative gynecology. He is also the chief medical officer of Vayas Health, a start-up technology company designed to provide the latest health information to health care consumers and physician offices. He is the author of *The Whole Pregnancy Handbook* and the medical director of the Association for Prenatal and Perinatal Psychology and Health.

Here, Dr. Evans talks about how our spiritual selves can support our health and overall well-being.

The mind and the body are connected through every major organ system. If the connections are unhealthy ones, then the body will not be in a state of optimal health and cannot truly heal. That's why it's important to use multiple modalities to understand patients' underlying emotional and spiritual issues to help them on their path to healing. That's what I do, and it starts with a conversation that ensures a patient knows she's heard and understood. We look at all the components of health—for example the diet, hormonal imbalances, and mitochondria health, which affects mood and neurodegenerative disease. We use state-of-the-art Western medicine to treat any medical issues, and we combine it with the wisdom and holistic approach of Eastern medicine. However, we also address physical imbalances and disease by working on stress through spiritual methods.

The importance of spirituality in health and healing is something that can't be over-emphasized. People are feeling disconnected from their life's purpose. That can result in a feeling of being untethered, of being not in your sweet spot in life, and that in turn creates stress on the body. *Allostatic load* is the fancy term for this disconnection, and it can cause the body to break down in many different ways. It exacerbates chronic conditions. Some people break down in their stomach areas and digestion; others get headaches.

It's time to embrace that. If you are going to go on a journey to health, you must do whatever you can to help your body heal and work better. Part of that process is taking away the thoughts, feelings, and emotions that hurt your physical body. The way you take away those thoughts, feelings, and emotions is first by understanding that you are not your physical illness. When you think peaceful, loving, and happy thoughts, your body is flooded with chemicals that make you feel healthy and happy. If you think thoughts that are stressful or that make you sad or depressed, then your physical body won't feel good. It won't heal as quickly.

If you have been diagnosed with a chronic illness, you have to be especially concerned about stress on the body. You also have to be very aware of your emotional and spiritual state. First, know you are more than your physical body. *You are not your illness.* For example, you may be a person who happens to have colitis, but you are not colitis. That's not what defines who you are. When you distance yourself from your illness in this way, you realize that there is a part of you that has no illness. Think about it: If you close your eyes and imagine that you lost your arm, would you still be yourself? Of course you would be. If you lost two of your arms, would you be yourself? Of course you would be. Likewise, if you happen to have a chronic health condition, you are still yourself aside from and separate from that illness. There's a lot about you that's right.

Realizing you're more than your physical body is so freeing and liberating. Your physical body is a part of you, but it's not what defines you. This understanding makes it easier to do what has to be done in order to maximize the likelihood that your body will heal. ■

Start Where You Are

How we start our day is essential to making it a good one. If you have time to make coffee and watch the morning bad-news channel, you definitely have ten minutes to meditate and set yourself up for a successful day.

If you don't give yourself time to start your day from a place of peace, then I guarantee it's going to be one hell of a twenty-four hours. If you start your day with chaos, you will have a chaotic day, *all* day. So wake up, sleepy head, and do some light stretches. Put your phone in a drawer, sit your body up, and practice one of this book's breathing exercises or do a body scan to connect with yourself before you run off to the doc, or the acupuncturist, or the office. You can set your alarm to go off ten minutes earlier than usual to give your body and mind the time to start your day from a place of peace and ease.

Take a Time Out

Our mind moves a mile a minute. I can literally think about at least fifteen things consciously all at once. It isn't easy being inside this head of mine. If you are like me, you could be planning a get-together, reminding yourself to pay your insurance bill, thinking about what shoes you want to order from ShopBop, mulling over how cute the boy two seats down from you on the subway is, wishing that your sister would apologize for the shitty thing she said to you earlier, and contemplating what you may want to snack on later that afternoon—all simultaneously. Just thinking about *thinking* that much and that fast makes me feel tired. There is no room for peace at this speed. So cool it, sis. Give yourself five glorious, uninterrupted, luxurious minutes to slow down your speedster mind.

First, sit down. Find something comfy—a cushion, pillow, couch, bed, or pile of blankets. Put your phone on airplane mode.

Next, choose something in your space that you can focus on and that brings you comfort. Beginners often choose to light a candle and focus on the flame. You can also choose something else, such as a little statue or a vase of flowers or whatever you like. It's yours and yours alone for the next five minutes.

Begin to scan your body for any discomfort. Let your mind go to any places that feel uneasy. Don't try to control or change the discomfort; just acknowledge that it's there with love and sit with it. Bring your attention to that place. Don't judge it. Just allow yourself to be with it and feel it. And breathe. Breathe into the place of discomfort without judgment.

Now try to drop those fifteen-mile-an-hour thoughts and see how many inhales and exhales you can get to without *one* stressful thought popping in. Try to get to ten, in and out. I dare you to try! You know how we do squats so that our tush looks good? Commit to breathing this way like you commit to doing to your squats because it makes your inside feel good, and your outside will thank your inside later.

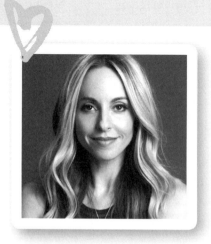

Gabrielle Bernstein

Gabrielle Bernstein has been named "a new thought leader" by Oprah Winfrey. She appears regularly as an expert on *The Dr. Oz Show* and was named "a new role model" by the *New York Times*. Gabrielle recently teamed up with Deepak Chopra to co-host the *Guinness Book of World Records* largest group meditation. Gabrielle is the *New York Times* bestselling author of the books *May Cause Miracles* and *Miracles Now*. Her other titles include *Add More ~ing to Your Life* and *Spirit Junkie*. In 2016 she will release her fifth book, *The Universe Has Your Back*.

YouTube named Gabrielle one of sixteen "YouTube Next Vloggers"; she was named one of Mashable's "11 Must-Follow Twitter Accounts for Daily Inspiration" and was featured on the *Forbes* list of "20 Best-Branded Women on Twitter." She has been featured in media outlets such as *ELLE*, OWN, *Kathy Lee & Hoda*, *The Today Show*, *Oprah's Super Soul Sunday*, *The Queen Latifah Show*, *Anderson Live*, *Access Hollywood*, *Marie Claire*, *Health*, *SELF*, *Women's Health*, *Glamour*, *Help Desk*, the cover of *Experience Life* magazine, and more. ▶

Gabrielle is a certified Kundalini yoga and meditation teacher. She is also trained in the Emotional Freedom Technique (EFT), and she's a student of Transcendental Meditation (as taught by the David Lynch Foundation).

Here, Gabrielle gives us insight into how our illnesses are connected to a disconnection from the spiritual aspects of our lives.

I have always been of the mindset, as a meta-physician, that the root cause of our physical condition is our spiritual condition. Every physical illness has a root cause—a disconnect from the spiritual or the connection to love. For many of us, this disconnect happens during a childhood detour into fear. Even the tiniest idea that the world is a fearful place can separate us from the loving presence we actually are. Once we go on that detour, we build a world around it, and that fear begins to take over in certain areas of our bodies.

Of course, we have to work through all the steps of physical healing when we're sick. We have to take the right medicine and follow the right guidance. But without the spiritual aspect of ourselves taken good care of, we can delay or stall true healing. We always have to heal the root condition, our spiritual condition, as part of the overall strategy to be well.

It's so simple to get in tune with your spiritual self. A daily practice of meditation and prayer opens our consciousness to other possibilities of support. We are more open to receiving spiritual guidance; it raises our awareness and consciousness, and it helps natural healing take place. Prayer and meditation go in hand-in-hand with relaxation, and you can expect tremendous healing benefits.

The first step is to want to heal and to set an intention in that direction—as in, "I am willing to heal spiritually." Or, "I intend to heal the root cause of my pain. I don't know how that will happen, but that's my intention." Setting that intention is like opening an invisible door. Intentions have to come from your own desire. Once you've set that intention, pray for it to be realized. You can trust you will be guided to the next right action.

Then be very present in the moment and pay attention. Guidance will come from your medical doctors, but also from other teachers that show up in any form: the book that's been sitting on your shelf for a while or something that happens in your yoga class. Once you invite consciousness in, you will hear and see guidance in all sorts of unexpected places. Invite it in, witness it, and act on the messages and the wisdom you're receiving.

Meditate every day for just five minutes—and longer if you can. But I promise just five minutes will make a difference in your day. I pray in the morning and in the evening, and I recommend you try it as well. When I am out and about, I am in active meditation in that I'm mindful of where my energy is going. If I sense I am out of alignment with my positive and powerful feelings of connectedness, I use conscious breathing to come back home. These are such simple practices anyone can do; they fit into everyone's day.

I am a big believer in keeping my spiritual reminders out so I see them and use them. It can be a small altar on the tabletop in your room where you place meaningful objects. I keep many crystals on my home altar and on my work desk. The crystals hold energy that inspires me and ignites freedom from the pain. I use what I call a God Box, in which I place my intentions and prayers. Writing down prayers and then putting them in such a box and trusting they are being taken care of is powerful. Consider placing prayer notes around your house as gentle reminders. Write down your intentions and pin them to a vision board or on your bathroom wall, or tape them to your computer. The idea is to have them visible so you can interact with them.

There are two meditations I want to tell you about. Both of them are from my book *Miracles Now* and come from Yogi Bhajan, who brought Kundalini yoga to the West in 1968. The first is the "Peace Begins With Me" meditation. This is such a great meditation

for releasing anger and resentment—something that people with chronic conditions often feel toward themselves.

Gently press your thumb against your index finger, then your middle finger, then your ring finger, and then your pinkie finger.

When you touch your index finger, say: PEACE.

When you touch your middle finger, say: BEGINS.

When you touch your ring finger, say, WITH.

When you touch your pinkie finger, say, ME.

Breathe deeply as you say each word.

You can do this meditation as quickly or as slowly as you like. And the great thing about it is that you can say the words silently to yourself—meaning you can say this meditation while you're waiting in the doctor's office, dealing with nosy co-workers, or even your own emotions as they are pressing down on your soul.

The "Meditation to Prevent Freaking Out" is the second one I recommend. It's a ▶

▶ very effective way to stop a freak-out before it begins.

POSE: Sit comfortably in Easy Pose (cross-legged) with your spine straight.

HANDS: Interlace your fingers with your right thumb on top. Place your hands at the center of your diaphragm, lightly touching your body.

EYES: Gently close your eyes.

BREATH: Concentrate on your breath, bringing awareness to the tips of your nostrils. Notice which nostril is dominant right now. It may take a few moments to clarify the dominant nostril. Once you are aware of the dominant nostril, focus your attention on switching sides. Keep your shoulders down and relaxed. You can have pressure in your hands but none in your shoulders.

Continue changing the dominant nostril breath back and forth as long as you like.

Use this meditation whenever you need to prevent a freak-out. It's also a great one to teach young children. This easy practice will be a powerful tool for them to carry into their future. ■

Meditate

When I got serious about meditation, I signed up for a Vedic meditation course in New York City. I was full of anticipation and a little nervous when I walked into the class. The teacher was a beautiful redhead with a smile that beamed sunshine. She glowed from the inside out. Happiness seemed to flood her pores. My inner cynic looked her up and down and thought, "She can't really be *that* happy."

I remember staring at her for a few moments, watching her closely, and thinking, *Hmmm, well, if it's real, I may as well give meditation a try, because I want some of* that. Still uncertain of what "that" was, I learned to meditate.

The teacher gave me my own mantra. Awesome! Then it was time to sit in stillness. Being the type-A personality that I am, I sat myself upright on my meditation cushion, crossed my legs, shut my eyes, put my hands in a lotus position, and was totally psyched to be off to the races meditating. "Inhale, exhale? I got this."

Within seconds, sitting in stillness and just simply breathing felt torturous. I wanted to do an army crawl off the cushion and out the door. I peeked through my closed eyelids to see if this was a possibility and saw that the teacher's eyes were open as she was teaching the class. I sighed. "Well, there goes that idea."

Next I tried to think "let" on the inhale and "go" on the exhale. *Let go*—simple. Then the song from *Frozen* got stuck in my head. *Let it go! Let it gooooo!* Rats. Where did my mantra go? I was supposed to be thinking about my mantra, not Elsa and her icy powers.

At that time in my healing journey, it was painful to feel so uneasy in my skin, but I knew, deep down inside, that silence and stillness would provide me with a deeper look and connection to what was inside of me, who I was, and what I needed. So I committed to doing a meditation every day. It took a lot of commitment and dedication and a big sense of humor for my type-A alter ego to stick with it. All type-A Amy wanted to do was get her daily meditation time done and over with and move on to her next appointment. Stillness whooped my ass all over Manhattan and back again. Until it didn't. And then it felt divine. Just like that. Practice is a ritual in itself.

"I was raised Catholic. Catholicism never resonated with me, but I was interested in spirituality. I was interested in what was going on beneath the surface, and I was interested in Eastern religion. Buddhist philosophy made a lot of sense to me; it acknowledged suffering, and, having RA, I am very sensitive and keenly aware of suffering. Buddhism says you can have pain, but you do not have to suffer because of it. It was a completely new way of relating to pain, and it changed the way I experienced pain. I started meditating quite regularly. When I started practicing, many things started to shift, and my mind and body became a home for me."

Kaitlyn Lennon

Meditation is the best gift I have ever given myself. It is now my daily ritual. It gives me the chance to start every day from a place of peace and deep connection to myself. It grounds me and keeps me connected to my inner compass. Just because our physical circumstances happen to be scary and uncomfortable, it doesn't mean we need to live from that place of fear and discomfort. I moved out of that house a long time ago, and I am never going back. Everything feels better when we go within ourselves and connect with our inner guide. Doing so takes us out of fear and brings us back to love. When we have *tune-in time,* we arm ourselves to live an awesome life, filled with love and positivity and connection. We can then approach the day and its obstacles with ease. We can begin to see the world through rose-colored glasses because we choose to. This is a much better place to wake up and live in.

▼ ▼ ▼

I have a six-year-old niece, and we like to talk about the color pink and all things girly. We don't live near each other, but FaceTime allows us to connect as often as possible. During one recent session, she said to me, "I wish I could just hop through the phone and onto your big fluffy pillow so we could cuddle, don't you?" And I said, "Yes! I would love that!" Without even blinking, her reply was straight to the point, "I'm working on it."

I smiled with a questioning face as if to say, "How?" My niece said with complete conviction, "I've been working on an invention where I can press a button on the phone and you can come over and play. When we're done, I can press the button again, and you get home safely. What do you think?"

I stopped and took a deep breath and grinned from ear to ear. "I think that sounds amazing," I said.

A child has the beautiful ability to see all things as possible, with no ifs, ands, or buts, and from an uninterrupted place of joy. As we grow into adults, many of us lose our belief in what's possible. The goal of spirituality, especially for someone with chronic health issues, is to get back to this place of wonder, hope, and an unwavering belief in what's possible. Even if we can't foresee an invention coming to fruition, we can have the conviction to make our circumstances greatly different than how they are now.

When we begin our new mindful life, we begin to understand the concept that healing is a process and not a destination. Your body has not abandoned you. By finding a spiritual mindful practice, you can begin to embrace the idea that your physical body is only a part of you, and that you are embarking on a journey to do whatever you can possibly do to heal your physical body while consciously removing the thought patterns that hinder your healing. We have the conviction to lead our lives from a different space—a space of *yes,* where our reality, no matter what our diagnosis, is better tomorrow than it is today. Believe in the possible.

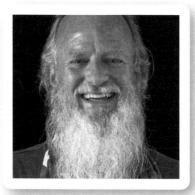

Thom Knoles

Thom Knoles is a maharishi or preeminent master teacher of Vedic meditation. He is a thought leader and celebrated speaker on the cognitive sciences, the potential of the brain, and the health of the body.

Here, Thom talks about how Vedic meditation can greatly enhance our quality of life and significantly help in the healing process.

Vedic meditation is a simple, natural, innocent, and effortless mental technique. It requires minimal time, about twenty minutes twice a day, and it's a delightful and high-impact experience. You notice the effect of it right away. It involves no special concentration or control. Once you've learned it, you just can't wait to do it again, rather than thinking, *Oh, it's a chore, and I've got to do this thing.* You close your eyes, and you make use of a little sound that you learn in the form of a word called a mantra. It's a specific mantra that is designed specifically for your use. Different mantras work best for different people.

Vedic meditation does come from ancient India, but it's free of the mystical trappings. It doesn't have cultural challenges. You don't have to wear any unusual clothing, you don't have to change your diet, and you don't get a new strange name that you have to announce to your family at Thanksgiving.

Overall, the preference is to sit upright while meditating because sitting upright keeps us in the least-excited waking state. If we lie down in order to meditate, we are likely to fall asleep, and we don't want to do that. Falling asleep is a good thing, but meditation is far more restful than sleep. So to get that maximum impact, we want to meditate sitting upright comfortably, with our back supported. We just close our eyes, sitting comfortably upright on a chair or a couch, or on the floor against a wall with pillows behind our back and head.

When you close your eyes and use your mantra effortlessly, the mind settles down to its least-excited state. And the body follows into a state of restfulness that is many times more restful than sleep. Consequently, when you come out of meditation, you feel ▸

▶ fantastic. During meditation, all kinds of wonderful effects are had due to its restfulness. The body is able to release and relieve existing accumulated stresses, and you are able to adapt outside of meditation to not become so easily stressed.

This de-stressing through meditation is so important for someone with a chronic condition because stress makes all conditions worse. Today's mind is printing out tomorrow's body. By that I mean that the number one governing effect on the body is the way the mind works. Peptides and proteins, neurotransmitters, transmit to the body the instructions from the brain as to how the body should behave. If I think an angry thought, then within seconds I have angry molecules all over my body. If I have an experience of sadness, within ten minutes the chemical structure of my body has utterly altered itself into a bag of sadness chemicals. An experience of fear will flood the body with fear molecules. The effect of the feelings you have today will create what you are tomorrow.

When we find ourselves mired in a condition, we have to release stress from our body because we know that stress makes every condition worse. There is no condition that is not made worse by stress. From the simplest kind of disease, like migraine headaches, to

very complicated, high-impact diseases, like HIV or AIDS, all symptoms are made worse by stress. If we can remove stress, we simplify what the disease condition is, and we make it easier to actually see what we need to target. Second, we remove all of the frustration that the body has in attempting to heal.

As you practice meditation, you will find yourself to be less stressed out outside of meditation. You will also find it easier to reduce stress in such situations that may have caused it in the past, before you had a meditation practice. As a bonus, you will occasionally have deep experiences of feeling at one with everything around you during meditations. This experience is a sign that you are in the least-excited-mindset state. This is bliss. The chemistry of bliss and the chemistry of healing happen to be identical. The more often we can have a bliss experience during meditation, the more quickly we can heal. We can accelerate that state by reminding ourselves from time to time, "I am one with the totality of nature's intelligence. I am one with totality. I am totality."

If I am one with all of that, the mentality of that is metabolized—that is to say, I metabolize the positive effect of that thought. I ingest it. That mindset works much better for someone who is having that experience through meditation than for them to think that thought when they haven't yet had the meditation experience. But it is helpful for us to have expansive and inclusive thoughts anytime, whether we have learned to meditate or we haven't yet learned to meditate.

There is scientific evidence for the skeptics out there, and it's quite powerful. In 1982 the *International Journal of Neuroscience* published a study entitled "Reversal of Aging in People Who Practice Meditation." In the study, four thousand policyholders with Blue Cross Blue Shield had their body ages measured.

When you measure somebody's body age, you may find a thirty-year-old whose body age measures as thirty-five or even forty if they have been a little disrespectful to their body or they have been diseased. If they have been very respectful to their body, the thirty-year-old might have a body age of, say, twenty-five or twenty-six. We have a chronological age, and we have a body age as well. There is a way of measuring body age called "Morgan's Adult Growth Examination Index." When we apply that index to the body, an algorithmic computer program reveals a body age, which can be older or younger than how many birthdays a person's had. It's rare that it's exactly the same as the chronological age.

Every one of those four thousand policyholders with Blue Cross had their body ages

measured. The group was randomly divided into two. The first half learned meditation, and they practiced it for the next five years. The other half, the control group, did nothing different in their lives for the next five years. At the end of the five-year study, everybody had body ages measured again. In the meditating group, the peoples' bodies on average were thirteen years younger than they should have been. So their biological age had gone backward thirteen years.

The control group of non-meditating people, not surprisingly, aged at the standard for the United States. U.S. citizens age faster than any other population on Earth due to stress and toxicity. Among those, New Yorkers age faster than any Americans, by the way. The non-meditating group aged at the U.S. average rate, which is 1.2 biological years of age for each birthday. So 1.2 years of biological age is added with each passing year for most Americans. Basically, the control group showed no change, which was predictable. The meditation group showed an astonishing change.

So unless you have learned to meditate, you haven't tried everything to heal. When we meditate, we remove distractions, and our body is able to really put its full attention on getting the healing done as quickly as possible. ∎

9

Social Studies

Those of us with a chronic health condition often don't show it on the outside. Unless someone is walking in your shoes, has walked your path before you, or is walking it beside you, they will never truly understand what you are going through. Anyone who has experienced illness or has gotten sick has had the experience of being an outcast. I certainly have. It's what naturally happens. Under these circumstances, interpersonal dynamics can get really tricky. Getting sick stirs the pot of all relationships and casts everyone into uncharted territory.

Let's face it: people are human. They react to things in both predictable and unpredictable ways. Your friends and your family don't quite know what to do or how to behave around you, the "sick person." You don't quite know what to do either. Friends, family, and partners—no one knows what to say or how to act, and some people don't know how to keep up a relationship that could be vastly different from the version it was when you were well.

I realize now that I spent a good amount of my childhood and adulthood seeing myself

as a victim of my circumstance. When I was fixed in this victim state, I wanted someone to save me instead of me saving myself. Through my work with Lauren Handel Zander and the Handel Method, I was able to see how my set of circumstances, my personal dynamics, and my dynamics with others were keeping me stuck in a fixed state, which kept me from truly healing. It wasn't until I understood how all of these things affected my present reality that my life started to shift.

Baby Amy

My parents and I were dealt a tricky card at the onset of my back pain, and we did the best we could with what we had. They were with me all the way. As a child, I really had no choice but to depend on my parents to help me navigate the health care landscape and to follow their lead on healing my physical pain. I held their opinion higher than mine because, let's face it, at fourteen, what did I know? It's natural. In fact, I thought everyone else's opinion was right, and mine was wrong (if I

"RA has a social impact. It's a running joke that I'm a flake socially. My illness is all but invisible; my hands have bumps, but other than that I look 'normal' and healthy. Internally I am battling this war, and my joints are killing me. I often feel foggy-headed because RA is total inflammation of the body, and this does affect your brain. This presents a bit of a struggle, because obviously there's a lot I want to do, and I am often too tired to even keep conversations rolling. If you mention the pain you're in, you feel like you're complaining or making excuses, and so it's a very weird, charged thing with regard to social life. You have to deal with knowing that other people, even your closest family and friends, don't *really* get it. That's where a lot of the struggle comes from."

Kaitlyn Lennon

even had an opinion). From age fourteen on, I went to everyone else for answers and solutions. I never grew up. I never, ever walked on my own two feet because my ailments started when I was so young. The reality is the onset of my back pain arrested my childhood and, as a consequence, my life. It kept me frozen in child mode for a long time.

Since I was actually quite sick when I moved back home to Philadelphia after my disastrous trip to Israel, my dependence on everyone to make every decision for me only grew stronger. The problem with being back in my childhood home with a major health crisis at age twenty-five was that it enabled and reinforced my total dependence on my parents. But I wasn't a child anymore. The more I began to understand that the need for approval of every last decision was actually part of my problem, the more I started letting go and growing up. My whole life I had thought from the outside in when the key to healing relationships, healing our health, and healing our life happens from the inside out. I was looking to everyone: my doctors, my parents, my friends, everyone to make decisions for me because my situation felt too overwhelming to deal with myself. I was stuck wanting someone to "fix it" so I could move on.

What was wrong wasn't how much I needed my dad and mom and everyone else in my life; it was how much I needed them versus how much I needed *me*. This was a revelation to me. I was stuck with the reality that I would be with myself for the rest of my life, and I had to either make that reality work and create a life for myself or stay in my old room, in my old bed, and get a cat for company. I realized I had been using my parents for their opinions instead of trying to figure out what *I* thought. I needed to ditch my codependent side and start to really learn how to listen to what my body needed. Baby Amy had to go; my severe situation demanded it, and that was a lesson in itself. In order to get well, I needed to understand this dynamic, get unstuck, ditch my need for approval on all things, and get my butt in the driver's seat.

Moving away from my childhood home forced me into a self-caretaking mode I wasn't used to. I had no choice but to take responsibility for my decisions and myself as I never had before. I asked myself what I needed and what was best for me. My body and I started becoming close in a way we had never been. My spirit and I reconnected, and I was able to begin trusting my intuition on all things. My spiritual renewal and my trusting of my intuition also improved and deepened my relationship with my parents and family.

Friend or Foe?

You've met several amazing women in this book, the Glow Warriors, and every one confirms that their wellness journey has made

> *Empathizing with others does not mean you have to hang out with sick chicks.*

> "*I* realized I could be human. Cancer humbled me and showed me it was okay to be vulnerable and take risks. I did not have to be so insecure anymore. I felt loved and accepted and cared for. It softened me."
>
> Paige Marmer

them more compassionate and empathetic. It is easier for them to walk in the shoes of someone who may be in pain or is suffering on any level. I have certainly had this experience—every single day. After going through the difficulties I did, including symptoms that were and are often physically painful, not to mention inconvenient and exhausting, I became much more aware of the struggles of other people and how those struggles might influence their behavior. My experience touched the place in my heart that wants nothing but the best for all beings. I want to be able to find and see the light in others, including the sick chicks.

Empathizing with others does not mean you have to hang out with sick chicks. It just means you wish them well and choose to help them via kind and loving thoughts. Eventually, they will find the compassion they need for themselves. As the popular saying goes (and it's quite true), "Kindness. It doesn't cost a damn thing. Sprinkle that shit everywhere." I want to find goodness in everyone. As you offer kindness, understanding, and goodwill to others, don't forget about yourself.

I was one of *those* people: I told everyone literally everything I was feeling. I complained constantly and dumped all of my baggage onto everyone I love. I likely was so annoying that people didn't want to speak to me or be in my presence. I was alienating myself because I simply wasn't conscious. It never once occurred to me to say to myself, "Wow, maybe I'm sending a really negative message into the world." I just wasn't that self-aware. I was so wrapped up in sick chick mode that complaining was as normal to me as washing my hands or brushing my teeth. I was leaking pain all over all of my relationships because the pills weren't helping my pain, the outside-in approach wasn't working, and I didn't understand that I needed to heal from the inside out, not the outside in.

However, in all honesty, many of my friends weren't real friends. Most of them were fair-weather friends. When tragedy happens, you learn who your people are. This is a gift. This is definitely what happened to me, even though I couldn't understand it at the time. I thought, *Oh, poor me* when I lost my so-called friends, when really, their departure was a blessing. Eventually I realized that some of the people I considered to be great friends really weren't all that great, and it made room

for me to find people who were. Lauren Handel Zander, in her coaching, called it "the Crucible Effect," and it occurs when something traumatic or significant happens in your life. And, in the face of that change, whether an illness or even something positive—like quitting drinking, losing weight, finding love—friends show their true colors. They fall short. They don't show up. They prefer you drunk. They offer a cookie. They disappear when you're sick. That's the crucible; when subjected to high "heat," certain friends melt away.

> The best thing you can do for the people you love is to ask for what you need and ask them what they need.

Naturally, there were friends whom I let loose from my life, and those who drifted away because I wasn't as much fun as I was (to them at least) before I was sick. That's okay. Friendships and social connections evolve all the time; the process just gets accelerated when you have a chronic condition that puts new demands on your schedule and on your well-being. Some of these are the same people who are skeptical about your symptoms and suffering, especially if the illness is not visible and you "look healthy," or if it hasn't been diagnosed with something recognizable, like the Big C.

What I once thought was a very large circle of good friends has become much smaller over the years. I've cleaned house. A chronic condition can toss a hand grenade into a lot of relationships, but it's also a good litmus test to show us who is really a friend and who isn't. When you have a chronic health condition, people aren't sure what to do, how to be there, or how to help. The best thing you can do for the people you love is to ask for what you need and ask them what they need. This supports you and them. Either they will show up or they won't.

I'd much rather have a small group of amazing people around me than a large group of disengaged people. The people who are there for you do not expect you to push yourself for them. These are the people to whom you can say, "Look, I'm too tired to go out or even sit and talk, but will you come and watch *Modern Family* with me?" and they'll do it. They may even be on their way without you asking. Those friends are real, and you are lucky to have them. When you have friends who fill you up and wrap you in love, do you need ten others who don't? I am grateful for having people like this in my life, and I make sure I let them know how much I love them as often as I can.

"Everything comes down to human connection for me and sharing fun activities with the people I love. I have come to realize the value and worth I have, which allows me to more deeply love the things that I involve myself in and the people I surround myself with."

Paige Marmer

You Are in Control

Just because you are dealing with a health condition doesn't mean you are off the hook when it comes to being a good friend, colleague, daughter, lover, spouse, sibling, and so on. You can't control other people, but you *can* set the tone and help them understand what you're going through and what you need and want from them. At the end of the day, they are going to behave and respond in their own way. However, you are 100 percent in charge of your responses to them. You're in the driver's seat. Stay in your own lane. You can turn around a lot of awkward situations by responding to people in appropriate and compassionate ways.

You can also try to set people up for success. Do this by exploring what you need and feel and want from each individual. The truth is you have a list of what you wish and really need from each individual person in order to have an amazing relationship with him or her. Setting expectations with everyone in your life is your job, and it's a wonderful opportunity to get clear on who you are and what you want and need. If you are taking care of your needs and doing what you can for the people you love, that's what's important.

Be part of the solution. Caution! Truth bomb ahead: people with chronic conditions sometimes alienate others because all they talk about is their ailments. (Cue Baby Amy! I used to be one of these people.) This goes all the way back to chapter 1 when we talked about putting an end to defining ourselves through our illness. If you talk about being sick all the time, you not only get sicker, but it also turns people off. Let's focus on telling the good stories and describing the great things that are happening to us so we can have a life and deal with our condition on the side.

There is no room for sitting and complaining when you are ditching fear and choosing love and the things that make your soul happy.

If we can't think of any good stories, that's a cue to us that we need to engage in something. Even if it's as small as knitting a scarf or doing an arts project at home. *Get a life.* Know your audience. Understand that people don't like complainers. If you need to talk about the bad feelings, go to your team of Glow Warriors or your therapist and/or coach, who can listen, empathize, and give advice when you are feeling low to help you accelerate into growth and action. There is no room for sitting and complaining when you are ditching fear and choosing love and the things that make your soul happy.

It's up to you. You need to ask for what you need and want. For example, "I know things are shifting a bit and my sickness is affecting our friendship. I'd love to see you once a month, but if that doesn't work, as long as you call me once a week, I'll know you love me regardless." Then give people the chance to show up. It's up to you if you want to keep the people who don't show up when they don't meet your expectations and needs. But you also have to reevaluate whether or not you're asking too much of people. In terms of friendships, I flushed a lot of the ones I didn't care about. I realized I was lost in interpretations of what other people thought, instead of asking myself what *I* thought. By doing this, I made room for new relationships, and cultivated the old ones that deeply mattered.

EXERCISE What Do You Need?

Now is the time to reassess and reevaluate your relationships. Are they all just the way you want them to be? Do you have the right relationships with the right people? It's up to you to understand and decide whom you need and what you want from each of your relationships.

Make a list. Be honest. Start with your family members and move on to friends, your partner, and your colleagues. Write down each person's name and write what kind of relationship you want with him or her. Start here:

Family

Who

What I need from them

What I can do for them

Take a critical look at the list. Is it honest? Is it realistic? How would you feel if these expectations weren't met?

✓ **EXERCISE** *What Do You Need?*

Friends

Who

_____

_____

_____

_____

What I need from them

_____

_____

_____

_____

What I can do for them

_____

_____

_____

_____

Colleagues

Who

What I need from them

What I can do for them

Partner

Who

What I need from them

What I can do for them

Others

Who

What I need from them

What I can do for them

Write On!

Writing is a very powerful resource. If you are struggling with getting clarity on an issue, if you have a great observation or thought, or if something is bothering you, you can jot down what comes into your mind. It's important not to judge what you have written, but instead look at writing as a way of understanding yourself more deeply. It puts you in a powerful position—a position of helping and healing yourself. You are present within yourself when you write. Getting your feelings out on a page is so good for you. So get yourself a journal and keep it by your side.

Get Help!

Ultimately, you need support from someone who doesn't judge you, has no emotional baggage *with you,* and can help you create an action-oriented plan around your condition. You aren't superwoman. It is totally natural to need to speak to someone about what is going on, and in my opinion it is 110 percent healthy. It is an amazing thing to be able to work through all of the feelings and emotions that come up when you're dealing with a chronic condition.

When I was looking for a therapist, I wanted someone who would be in a constant dialogue with me. I liked the idea of having someone who had worked with people that have struggled with their health before. I didn't want sympathy; I wanted to find the person who could help me make an action-oriented plan so I didn't feel helpless. I found that person, and it has powerfully transformed my health and my life.

A therapist or a coach is able to give you their undivided attention and unbiased opinion. Your mixed feelings and emotions that are bottled up inside of you are like an apple rotting on the counter. If you don't take out the trash, it's gonna start to stink, just like your life (your body, your mind, your condition) will if you don't get help. It is so natural and healthy for you to work with a professional to purge and process your feelings and come up with a plan that supports you. This person will be your partner in working through the reality of your situation. Choose wisely.

Howdy, Partner

Being sick and getting healthy can be tricky when you're in an intimate relationship. I've had to work very hard with my partner to establish a normal routine while going through my health journey. If I allowed myself, and I have certainly had my moments, Baby Amy could have just hopped right into an unhealthy dependent dynamic. Here's the deal: The same rules apply to all of your relationships, and they especially matter in this one. Treat them as your partner: be honest, share the good news and improvements and let them know what's not going great as well. You have to keep the relationship as normal as possible for them and for you. The minute your partner doesn't see you as whole, the relationship shifts in ways that aren't healthy. You're no longer equal, each putting in the same amount of care. An imbalance happens.

If you want to keep them on your team, you have to toss the ball back and forth: here is what you need; here is what I need. When you're not feeling up to something, instead of whining or pouting, say, "You know, I'm figuring out what I need right now, so it's okay for you to make your own plans this week." Or, "Maybe we can get a massage together next week." Let them have their own space. Be an active participant in suggesting activities that you both can enjoy based on what you feel you can do.

Think about how you can have fun, intimate time together outside of the health situation you're dealing with. This is crucial. When you do things with your partner, you get out of your shell and direct yourself outward and toward the other person. To help you and your partner create a life outside of your illness, consider these practical questions:

> "I try to be more vocal with my husband now. In the beginning [of my pain and foot issues], I wouldn't communicate the way I was feeling. Now I am much better at telling him that I have to sit down, I am in pain, or I am not feeling well. No complaints, just the truth. That has made the relationship better."
>
> *Morgan Segal*

▸ What are things you love to do together?

▸ When and how can you do them, or do them more often?

▸ What are new things you both want to try that are in the realm of your abilities?

▸ When can you plan them?

If you don't have a lot of energy, make sure you save time for your partner. Have weekly check-ins, so that your partner is on the same page and knows what's going on for you physically. The better your lines of communication are, the better your relationship will be. Your relationship with your partner is your most sacred relationship aside from the one you have with yourself. Honor and cherish your partner in the way he or she deserves.

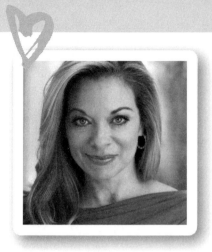

Terri Cole

Before earning a master's degree in clinical psychotherapy from New York University and adopting a lifestyle of daily meditation, green juice, and exercise, Terri Cole worked as a talent agent for actors and supermodels. When it became evident that the things (money, power, sexy job) she thought would make her happy didn't, she went back to school and became a licensed psychotherapist and built a successful practice. Terri is also the founder and CEO of Hello Freedom, a life coach, and a thought alchemist. A two-time cancer survivor, she specializes in helping people overcome the fear that can paralyze their lives.

Here, Terri shares her strategies for living fearlessly—so important when navigating the potential landmines of personal and family relationships.

At your diagnosis, there is fear and panic, that period of time when the new reality is sinking in. It's similar to the grieving process. You go through the same phases—shock and denial, pain and guilt, anger and bargaining, and depression—before getting back on track. Eventually, if you're adaptive, you can get to a place of reframing the experience for yourself. So many people in this situation want to revert back to an earlier phase, when things were good, or they think, *The doctors know what to do. I'm just going to do what they say.* You have to take ownership of the journey you are on, especially if it is chronic and long term. You have to ask, "How do I live well with this?"

MAKE AND IMPLEMENT A PLAN OF ACTION. Give yourself a period of time to grieve, but then you need to get your shit together. Do you want to pull yourself up and make a plan, or stay where you are? In the beginning, the fear is so intense you may feel you don't have control, but you do. You have to get busy. Do something creative with it. A friend of mine filmed her journey with cancer, and that created a buffer between her terror and mortality and made it okay. She put on her filmmaking hat and looked at dailies; it was absolutely terrifying. What if no one wanted to see a documentary about cancer? But she did it anyway. There is a clinical term for that, *adaptive functioning,* which refers to the skills necessary to effectively navigate the demands that are placed on us by our environments.

My plan was to become an expert on my cancer, and I did. Every study, every choice, East and West medicine—I knew it all. That enabled me to find my inner warrior and question the doctors. I went to the best person in the country; he was an extremely skilled surgeon and a complete asshole, a master-of-the-universe type. I actually ended up firing him and went to someone with a better bedside manner, who was also a skilled surgeon and, in fact, head of surgery at his hospital. There is always another option.

DON'T LET YOUR FEAR MIND RUN YOU. First you have to be present, which can be hard because a part of your mind will want to run away. Your fear mind can be so powerful; kick the crap out of fear mind. You have to realize you are not your fearful thoughts. Just because you have fearful thoughts, it does not make them true. Fear is projecting into the future about something that has yet to happen and may never happen. If you make a decision—"Oh, I'm going to die so I won't have treatment"—you're projecting into the future. You have to be able to recognize when your fear mind is telling you the terrible stuff. You have to be strong to slay your fear and make friends with your fear mind: "Hey, pal, you're not going anywhere until I'm dead. So why not be friends?"

CREATE AWARENESS. The number one thing I do with clients is guided visualization, which they can do while they are doing chemo or receiving any kind of treatment, or when their fear mind has a hardcore hold over them. Guided visualization is an amazing help for people who feel compromised. Harnessing the mind-blowing power of your own intention is more powerful than anything else you can do. Here's the thing: if you are to get better and own your life, mindfulness—yes, being mindful—is the key. You cannot live in that swirl of fear because you are living in the future you are dreading. Worrying, projecting fearfully into the future, is praying for the exact opposite of your desired outcome, so you don't want to do that. You have to have the courage to use your power for good.

BE MINDFUL OF WHAT TRIGGERS YOUR FIGHT-OR-FLIGHT REACTION. You can absolutely stop, but you have to be present. You can't think about what might happen in the future or ruminate about the past. There is only one moment of time you can be in, and that's now. When I start flipping out, I feel a constriction in my chest, but it's different for everyone. I use a simple fear exercise. When you are present, you think, *Oh, I don't have to flip out. I am going to locate where that constriction happens, and I am going to close my eyes, and I will breathe and send that ball of crap on its way and* ▶

▶ *explode it into a million pieces. And then I'm going to replace that shit with something that is empowering.* Think of someone you love, a child you love, or say to yourself, "Hey, everything is fine. Just slow down your breath."

Consciously notice what's around you, which is a grounding technique. Instead of being a helium balloon with your feet off the ground, breathe and slow down your heart rate. I stop, push up against a building, breathe, and say to myself, "This wall behind me is cold. My feet are on the ground. I hear a taxi." It's a way of pulling yourself back to the present moment, so you can shift from fear to neutrality.

DON'T GIVE YOUR POWER TO SOMEONE ELSE. We come in alone, and we go out alone. That is the truth about life. If you are lucky enough to partner with someone, lucky you, but you are the only one who lives through the choices you make. You do not need to convince anyone of anything. When you try to do this, you lose your power.

I'm not saying don't share your struggle with friends or significant others. People say the dumbest shit ever, and it's so annoying. People don't know what to say. You have to be clear about the boundary. If you are not asking someone for a suggestion, and they give you unwanted advice or criticism, say, "I am not problem solving now. If you could just care that I'm in pain and hold that advice back for a while, that would be wonderful." This is a skill, one you have to develop.

Whether you have the most invisible or obvious illness, it kicks up people's shit. You have people who avoid you or burst into tears when they see you. I have a friend who burst into tears every time she saw me. "Oh my gosh, why are you crying? Are you okay?" Then I realized she was crying about my diagnosis, and I felt terrible, which made me want to say, "How is my having cancer about you all of a sudden?" As women we are the bridges, the socializers, and when you are the one who is always making sure everyone is okay, there is no space for you to be okay. You have to make that space and ask people for what you need and want. Friends say, "What can I do?" *You* have to tell them what you need.

You should absolutely be doing energy work; it's not as out there as it sounds. It works. Protect your energy with an Epsom salt bath at the end of the day; it will wash away all the negativity that might be out there. I sage my home often and especially after people leave my house. Before you leave the house or before you have a meeting, you can zip up your energy. It's a simple but very effective strategy. Take your hand, put it on your pelvic bone, and then draw it straight up to your mouth. Do this three times.

COMMUNICATE CLEARLY. You have to communicate honestly and without anger. If you have a friend who loves you and is flipping out, say, "Here's the thing, Betty. I have to take care of myself. I can't take care of you." You can talk to other people about your diagnosis, but if they're flipping you out, don't talk to them about it. Set your friends and family up for success; send a little email. If too many people are asking questions, send emails to update everyone as to where you're at, just as a way of not having to have that same conversation four hundred times. Be discerning about who is on the list and then say, "Hey, this is where I am at. If anyone wants to do something, here's what you can do." And then let them know specifically what they can do. You can train people, because if you leave them to their own devices, they will fail you.

SEEK HELP FROM AN IMPARTIAL EXPERT. Everyone needs someone to talk to who is impartial and is trained not to bring her baggage into the conversation. That can be a psychologist, coach, or social worker. One of the benefits of coaching is that you get support from someone who knows more about something than you do. They know how to work with strategies to deal with the fear. You want a therapist or coach who is speaking to your healthiest, most resilient self, teaching you how to access that self, and holding that very high place for you.

When interviewing potential therapists, go in with questions so you can find out if they are right for you. Remember, they are working for you, not the other way around. Interview them just like you would interview anyone else. Most coaches and therapists will give you a twenty-minute free consultation, so take it if it's offered. There are five easy questions. The first three are for you to ask the therapist; the last two you ask yourself:

1 Have you worked with someone who has what I have?

2 Are you an interactive therapist? Or do you do the Freudian thing and stare at me for forty-five minutes? (You probably want someone who interacts.)

3 Are you familiar with and do you have experience working with people who have chronic illness?

4 Do you like the therapist's vibe and their office?

5 Finally, do you like them? Do you feel a connection? ∎

"After a lot of deliberation, I decided I needed to tell my bosses about my MS. I travel a lot, and when I land at a different city airport, when I am walking across the airport, I get a rush of pins and needles. They needed to know. Once we were going to work with the Philadelphia Eagles, and I was so excited. I was going to meet the coach and interview some amazing people. I was so excited the morning of the meeting. I was getting ready, and my husband called a cab for me. All of a sudden I got very lightheaded and completely wiped out and was unable to stand up. This had never happened to me before. And I had to say I couldn't do it. My bosses were very understanding and have been so since I told them about my condition."

Lindsay White

Navigating Social Landmines

Here are my tips for handling the social combat zone with your closest friends and family when you have a chronic condition.

TIMING IS EVERYTHING. Don't drop a bombshell at the last minute when you're calling to cancel a plan. Give your friends and family some notice. Let people know what's going on, in an unemotional way, at an appropriate time.

DON'T GET ON THE WORRY TRAIN. Stop wondering what they'll think of you. I was on that ride for a long time, and it took me absolutely nowhere. The ones who can't handle your news will scurry away like mice. The ones who understand will stick with you.

ASK FOR WHAT YOU NEED. Always be honest. No one can read your mind! Instead of getting bratty and assuming people know what you need from them, put on your big-girl pants and simply say what you need: "You know, I'm feeling pooped right now. I think I need a nap." I spent a lot of time waiting for friends and my siblings to come to me while forgetting to let them know I needed them to. It put a lot of unnecessary strain on the relationship. I didn't clue anyone in and, in the process, set them up to fail! Totally uncool of me. Put both your mind and their minds at ease and tell your peeps exactly what you need when you need it.

LET PEOPLE IN. Include those you love in *your* plans, and show them that you want to spend time in their company. Make a plan based on how *you* feel, but do be proactive. Again, don't wait for people to come to you with a perfect event that suits your needs. That's just not going to happen, or happen very often. You still have to be a friend because friendship is a two-way street. How about, "I would really love to zone out and watch a reality TV marathon this Sunday. Want to do it together?" Or, "Hey, I'm feeling a little tired, but I was thinking it might be fun to do this arts-and-crafts project. Do you want to join me?"

SET UP BOUNDARIES. You can't talk to everyone about what is going on; it is simply too much. It keeps you living in a state of constant fear and sick chick mode, which is not where you want to be. It's also exhausting. Don't share everything. This doesn't mean hide or lie. How about, "I'm hanging in there; thanks for asking." Then quickly turn it around, and ask them how they are. Toss the ball back and change the subject. Protect yourself, warrior. Be polite about your boundaries and don't be a meany.

THERE'S NO NEED TO PLAY CATCH UP. Sometimes a random person from your past hears something about you, and all of a sudden out of left field, they're on the phone checking in. When a person you haven't seen since the fifth grade calls out of the blue to check in, you really don't owe them an hour-long description of your last ten doctor's appointments. They might feel guilt or just be curious. Who knows? It doesn't matter. It's nice of them to think of you, but you don't

need to go into your entire diagnosis and everything the doc told you at your last visit. A simple, "Thank you so much for thinking of me. That is very kind of you. My doctors are handling everything, and I'm in good hands," is sufficient. Even better, say, "Thank you for your thoughtfulness. I really appreciate it. I am hanging in there," and then change the subject. Keep it simple for you.

Work It

The decision or question of whether to tell your employers about your chronic condition, or how much to tell them, and when, is a big one. The answer is yes, tell them the truth. Your employer should see the experience you

"There are instances when I just really don't feel well enough to be in a social setting, and I'm totally okay with that. I'm really not one to feel like I'm missing out. When you stay present with yourself, you're exactly where you are meant to be. You should just be honest with those around you when you're not feeling well, and know that taking time off is the right thing for you and your needs."

Tara Sowlaty

are going through as strength and not weakness. There should never be fear around your place of work. If you can get the job done, there is no reason for you or your employer to be afraid. If an employer doesn't understand, find another job, with an employer who *does* understand. This is easier said than done, I understand. But remember, you can't be fired because you are in the CC Club, especially if you are getting the job done. Honesty is the best policy; there may come a time when you are asked to do something at work that you *can't* do, and if you have not told at least your boss about a chronic condition, what are you going to do then? You have put yourself in a very difficult position.

Lying is a tricky business. Not only does it challenge your recall skills ("Now wait a minute, did I tell Reilly I had a cold, or did I tell her I was hung over from the night before? I can't remember"), but it also puts you in the awkward position of pretending to be someone you are not. Lying takes up energy that you need. A Glow Warrior can be honest with her boss, give her the 411 on her health, and let her know that the job will get done.

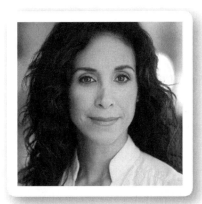

Lauren Handel Zander

Lauren Handel Zander is the cofounder and chairwoman of Handel Group®, an international corporate consulting and private coaching company and creator of the Handel Method®. The Handel Method®, which Lauren developed at MIT, is a step-by-step coaching process that addresses one's entire life and teaches people how to dream, how to realize their dreams, and how to clean out their closets (literal and figurative) so they can have lives of which they are wildly proud. The Handel Method® has been taught in over thirty-five educational programs, universities, and institutes of learning across the country, including MIT, Stanford Graduate School of Business and Stanford Medical School, New York University, Columbia,

Yale School of Drama, Wesleyan, Fordham, Rutgers, Barnard, Middlebury College, Scripps Research Institute, and in the New York City Public School System.

Here, she talks about honesty and keeping your own promises as a way to maintain sane and healthy relationships—so important when you're in the CC Club.

I am going to tell you the truth: your health is a lesson, and it is teaching you something important. It is showing you who your real friends are, so be prepared to learn the truth about everyone. When something serious and real happens to us, it allows people to step up or not, to show their true colors, even if their true colors make them jerks. It's also an opportunity to find out a lot about yourself. Being human is an amazing privilege—one we're not always really good at. There's so much knowledge and information in the world, and yet no one teaches us the really important things, like how to deal with a personal crisis or how to deal, aside from medical advice, with a serious or chronic illness.

In the face of illness, if you opt to see yourself only as the victim of it, your body just screws with you even more. The way you talk about yourself is creating your current reality. So, when you say, "I am sick," it's almost as if you are commanding yourself to be sick and for others to see you that way. Specific behavior follows. It's similar to when I ask people their life stories, and they accent the negative—where they suffered and at whose hands—which just perpetuates more negativity. When you say, "I am getting well," you are contributing to healing yourself. When you tell your life story using a positive narrative or positive examples, you're making a shift and shifting your relationships and how others hear and perceive you. I am getting you to think the right thing, and the right thing is you are the cure. This is part of what I call *Daily Design,* or *DD.* It's consciously creating your day, versus just having a day and seeing how it goes. This is putting the steering wheel back in your hands, making you the driver, the author of your own life, and not the passenger or the victim of any of it. By committing to designing your day, each day, it also allows you to practice making a promise to yourself and keeping it, daily. It's what I call *Personal Integrity,* where your actions (designing your day) align with your dream. In this case, your dream, your vision, is to be happy and healthy.

When dealing with yourself and how to fully believe in the reality of your vision, your desired state, you have to first deal with your current state. Start with reality versus the vision or the dream. What's the truth about where you are, compared with where you want to be and what that really looks like? ▶

Be honest. Don't lie to yourself; it makes you sicker. Then explain why you tell yourself you can't have the vision. Why are you stuck where you are? Because you're sick? Your answer is a thumbprint of how you think, and how you get stuck. Even though your current reality feels terrible, the unknown just seems worse. When you don't trust yourself, you give the illness a lot of power. It's thinking, *I'm stuck in my body,* versus *My body is trying to get me to wake up.* That's part of the lesson that the condition is teaching you. It's telling you to wake up about your friends and about authoring and designing your own life.

One way to do this is to design your day: "I'm going to be healthy and happy today" or whatever gets you closer to your dream. Then, you can assess whether a particular choice is in line with the vision. The vision tells you if you can or should do something. It tells you if you should make a change in a relationship or how you should be reacting to the people around you. That's why you have to do a DD every day. Personally, if I don't do my own DD by 10 a.m., I owe $10 to my women's group pot every time I miss one. It's what I call a *Consequence.* For each promise I make, I impose my own consequence, whether it's losing an episode of "Game of Thrones" (permanently!) or owing money to the political candidate I loathe most. It has me keep my promise or pay up, trumping any sort of feeling bad or need for an excuse. Guess what? More often than not, I keep that promise.

I have coached people through being sick, and the biggest mistake they can make is keeping it all a secret. I coached a woman with cancer, and she enlisted her husband in the lie to not to tell certain family members about it. When she came to me for coaching, she was a mess. It was killing her. She hated her job, and her relationships were in shambles. What was her vision? To be happy in her relationships and to have a better career. In order for her to make the vision a reality, she had to right those relationships. The lies were an obvious sign that something was deeply wrong with her relationships. This wasn't her first lie. She lied all the time. In order to get unstuck, she had to fix all of her relationships; otherwise, she'd never be healthy or happy again. And she had to stop lying.

To talk about your chronic condition effectively is when you can actually take responsibility for it. "But, I don't want people feeling sorry for me," is a common excuse people use to not speak about their illness openly. The lie, however, hurts everyone more. It keeps you from recharging. It keeps you small and the illness at the helm. Instead, say, "I am proud of my great attitude. I am choosing to bring love and healing to every moment." ■

10

Smile! You're a Glow Warrior!

Congratulations! You're a Glow Warrior, and now you know how to own it and show it to the world. As a Glow Warrior, you have the opportunity to set an amazing example for others through your behavior, demeanor, compassion, and health-loving vigor and happiness. Like you, I am still learning how to fully let go of my eleven years of chronic pain and live in the present moment. I am still on my own healing journey. But I have come so far using the tools in this book: I no longer need IVs five days a week, daily vitamin shots, an oxygen tank to breathe, or fifteen-plus hours of sleep to feel partially human anymore. My back pain is completely gone. I can enjoy food again, my thyroid is stable, my heavy-metal count is down, and the parasites are gone (bye-bye fuckers).

I no longer need everyone's opinion just to stand on my own two feet and make a medical decision. I have broken my addiction with codependency. I went from having a total emotional, spiritual, and physical breakup with myself at fourteen to being committed to loving myself into wholeness. I have deeply

healed my life. So while I'm still in the midst of healing my motility disorder, I choose to stay in the present moment and see how magical life really is, every single day.

Over the past six years I have experienced more shifts, changes, and challenges than I ever thought possible. I did all of that. I am a survivor. And now, I am a Glow Warrior. My own success tells me it will be no different for you. I know you can do it. By *living* the tools you have learned, and by smiling, engaging, and sharing what you know about health and wellness, you can do an incredible amount of Glow Warrior wellness work. You've gotten yourself connected to the glow within you and can live your life from that place now.

You've learned that it's possible to respect your own limits and make your needs clear with loving-kindness. Now you have to implement the things you've learned. My hope is that you will return to this book again and again for motivation, inspiration, and information.

Don't forget: you are so much more than your physical ailments. Embrace the fact that you are on a journey to do whatever you can to help your physical body work better and heal. Your body is only a part of what you are now committing to take care of and helping to heal. Healing is a journey, not a destination. It's time to get in the river and flow.

To send you off and set you up for success, I have created a kicking sick checklist. It includes many of the important topics we covered together, but I have written it as an action plan—a kick-start to kicking sick, if you will. Tackle one action step at a time, and you will see many benefits and positive changes—I guarantee it. Start where you are, and start right now!

The Kicking Sick Action Plan

The idea of the Kicking Sick Action Plan is not to tackle an action, complete it in a day, and forget about it. It is to initiate behaviors and activities that you can take with you on the journey to being healed.

Note that this isn't a twelve-day action plan, but a twelve-*part* plan. You can start at the beginning and work your way through all twelve parts in order, or you can start with the parts that mean the most to you and go from there. Take as much time as you need to practice each part. At the very end of this chapter is a journal to help you track your progress; it's a place to write down which

part you incorporated and how it made you feel. Writing things down is an affirmation; it makes your progress real and reminds you how much you've accomplished.

1 REMIND YOURSELF OF
YOUR TRUE IDENTITY

Today you will give yourself a tender reminder that you are exactly where you need to be at this moment. Today you will recognize that you are a beautiful, whole person. Today you will reframe any negative mindsets that you may have around your chronic condition.

Put your hand on your heart and feel it beating. That's you—you are alive! Take a deep breath. Begin the journey with your mantras, and make them part of your daily routine. Write some of the mantras on notes and put them where you will see them every single day: on your planner, your electronic devices, or your mirror. Post them all over your home. Set up your mobile phone to send you the mantra in a reminder message each day, at least once a day. The more you see them, the more you will start to believe what they say. Here are some example mantras for you to steal:

▸ With every breath I take, I am healthy, happy, and well.

▸ Perfect health is my divine right. I claim it now.

- All the cells in my body are vibrating with radiant health.

- I honor my body and its wisdom.

- I choose to be healthy.

- Each cell in my body is moving toward radiant health.

- I am full of good health and great energy. My mind is peaceful and calm.

- I am totality.

- I am a warrior. My strength is unlimited.

- Every single day I am getting healthier and stronger.

- I am whole.

- My cells are radiating with vibrant health.

- Every day I am getting better and stronger.

- I am glowing with good health.

- I am (your name). I am not (your chronic condition).

- I am (write your own new positive descriptor).

Write out your dream for the day, the week, the month. The minute you have a clear idea of what your true wish is, you reset the whole calibration of everything. You can stop and ask yourself at every step along the way, "Does this action (or decision, thought, or plan) align with my dream? Does this help get me to where I want to go?" Then you can sit with your intuition. Those of us in the CC Club have to be aware when our intuition feeds us fear-based thoughts. Once we get into a more present state and create a real dream for our healing, we are able to more clearly tap into what is right for us. Start to dream about your healing, how you want it to go, who you want to support you on the journey, and where you want to be in a week, a month, a year.

2 SET YOURSELF UP FOR SUCCESS
Today you take care of business. What do you need to be successful going forward? Get organized, my pretties. Dedicate this day to getting it together: Gather all your medical files, and put them on a thumb drive that you can keep in your bag. Round up copies of any X-rays, CAT scans, MRIs, doctor's notes, documentation, paperwork, lab results, and insurance info, and put it all in one place for easy access. You won't believe how getting organized reduces stress and anxiety. It's more satisfying than organizing your sock drawer. Organizing your information really *does* reduce stress. You'll be ready for the races in a

productive and healthy way. It's so important to make this space for yourself and get clarity about your medical history—especially since you're about to get your A-team together.

3 SET UP YOUR A-TEAM

Use my tools in chapter 4 to get your A-team together. Who are your health care providers? Go down the list. Which ones are serving you well, and which ones make you feel uneasy? Make sure the people who you are paying to help you heal give you what you need. If they're not, have the courage to ask for what you need or simply move on. These people work for you, so you decide who stays and who goes. Go through your top docs, healers, gurus, meditation teachers, and so on. While making your team, always check back in on your requirements for ideal doctors and other providers, and make sure you are choosing people who align with what you truly want for yourself and your healing. Who do you want on your A-team, and who goes off the list? Always be proactive and reassess the list when necessary. Never stop being a wellness activist and advocate for yourself. Make a list of the people on your team, and organize them into a list on a Microsoft Word document on your computer. Have their email, fax, and other info handy so you stress less when you are managing many people. Put that list on your mobile phone, your day planner, a notepad, and whatever else you use to organize your life.

4 CLEAN HOUSE

Today you will clean up your plate. What can you take off your plate that doesn't need to be there? What can you delegate to others? Take a good, long hard look at your life right now, and make the edits needed to get you to where you feel comfortable, a place where you're doing what you like to do and *not* doing anything that isn't serving you well. Every time you add something positive, get rid of something negative, including any pessimistic thoughts, a Debbie Downer attitude, or a tendency to scroll around the Internet late at night looking for a cure. Whatever it is that makes you feel bad, cut it out. Let it drop. Let it go.

5 PRACTICE SELF-CARE

Self-care is taking care of yourself in a tender, loving way every single day. Self-care is making sure you get what you need every day to thrive. What are the self-care rituals that help you the most? Aromatherapy? Have you tried tapping yet? How about dry brushing—getting your glow on with a nice, natural bristle body brush? Is your bedroom set up for a truly restorative night's sleep? Do you wake up gently and not to the piercing sound of an alarm clock? Do you allow yourself peaceful time in the morning, or are you off to the races, with stress all over you and around you? What can you shift and add in to your personal care rituals? What rituals can you make a part of your normal routine? Would a hot bath or regular naps serve you well? What about lying in savasana with cucumbers over your eyes? Need more downtime? How about carving out a time to engage your creativity—whether that's reading a good book, painting, gardening, or engaging in an arts-and-crafts project. Put on your pajamas and watch a comedy—and laugh, laugh, laugh.

Whatever it is that speaks to your soul, don't wait. Start now. Start adding the things that bring you joy, the more the better, and make them a regular part of your life. Pamper yourself every single day as you would someone you love, and do *at least* one thing that makes you truly happy as a person and that has nothing to do with your illness.

6 TAKE CARE OF HOME BASE— YOUR BOD

Clean out your kitchen. Assess what's on your shelves and in the fridge. Toss everything that you can't pronounce or that has an ingredient that makes no sense. Make a commitment to get rid of all the foods that are not serving you. Nourish yourself with a plant-based diet; fill the fridge with the colors of the rainbow and be a food detective! Refer to the list in chapter 6; print it out and take it to the store. Get rid of the crap and the junk. Make yourself a green juice or smoothie. Eat a salad. Fall in love with produce and fall out of love with bread and pasta. Choose one new healthy food that you can add into your daily routine. Swap the chips for a handful of healthy trail mix; swap the second cup of joe for a green juice. Small shifts equal big changes.

7 GET MOVING

Add exercise and movement to your daily routine. Start slow and small. Take a fifteen- or twenty-minute walk, and add five minutes to it each day. Try some simple hand-weight exercises and add in a few light yoga stretches, and voila, you have yourself a routine. Look for new activities to try: boxing, jumping, Pilates, dance. Take a class. Grab a buddy to keep you honest, and be accountable to each other. Then challenge yourself. Remember, you can always go just five minutes more. More often than not, your mind says no before your body does. Start from a place of joy and do something that makes you truly happy and free. Move it or lose it.

8 EXPAND YOUR RESOURCES

Become an expert on your condition. Keep learning, researching, and staying on top of the latest info about your condition. Reevaluate where you are: How do you feel? Do you need a change? Who can stay on your A-team, and who can join it? Find and add those wellness workers that enhance your life and health, and ditch the ones who don't. If a massage helps you feel better, schedule one immediately. If a vitamin drip gives you a boost, get it. If acupuncture helps relax you, by all means, make it a part of your health care and wellness habit. If you want to get your sweat on but find exercising too hard right now, go sit that cute tush in an infrared sauna and chill while you get your sweat on. Find a coach or therapist you can hash things out with, *without* judgment, and remember that your thoughts create your reality, so keeping them all locked inside is not serving you. Get it out so you can get on with it. Support yourself through the process. Your body will thank you later. Be your own best advocate.

9   CONNECT WITH YOUR HIGHER SELF

Do some soul searching. Go deep. Meditate. Remember, just five minutes a day can make a difference. That's *five minutes,* my friends! Surely you've got the time to quiet your mind and clear your head before plunging in to a busy day. Give yourself that quiet space where thoughts float by. If it helps, use a meditation tape, a guided meditation, or restful sounds of music. The goal is to connect with your inner self every day and commit to your loving inner self. When you feel outside of yourself, stressed from treatment plans, out of body, anything, go within. Remember: tune out to tune in. When you feel fearful thoughts, stop, drop, and breathe. The solution to staying in the present is always inside of you.

10   CREATE A TRIBE YOU LOVE

Mend relationships that matter, let go of destructive ones, and cultivate healthy new associations. It's essential to surround yourself with other Glow Warriors, as well as friends and family who are on your side, understand you, and make you feel supported and loved. Encircle yourself with people who feed your spirit and your mind. Who are they? Who are the people who show up for you the way you show up for them? Who are the people who care enough to make a new relationship with you and whom you care to make a new relationship with? If someone is not serving you well or is making demands you can't meet, you might have to slowly back away and break up. Wish them well and send loving-kindness their way, but move on. They aren't for you anymore, the way you once thought they were, and that is okay because it makes room for the amazing people who are. Don't worry about being lonely! When you are truly in touch with your authentic self, you attract like-minded people. The energy you give out from this new mindful place will attract people with that same energy back to you.

11   BE YOUR OWN BEST FRIEND

Take a good look at how you have been living your life up until now. Your thoughts and feelings are your reality. If you treat yourself like you would your bestie, you will be filled with loving-kindness and unconditional love.

Be kind to yourself. Slow down. Give yourself your presence. Now is the time to begin living with a new outlook. Forgive yourself. Choose to love again. Rise up into living life and approaching difficult situations differently. The time is now to thrive. The time is now to *rise* up. Life is yours for the taking.

12 SHARE THE GLOW

Put your best foot forward, share what you know with others, and give back. The goal of becoming a Glow Warrior is to optimize your well-being. A fabulous side effect of that is you become an ambassador of glowing health. Lead by example. Encourage others to follow your lead. How about writing a blog about your journey? Or starting a group where like-minded warriors get together to swap strategies and information? How about a cooking club that meets monthly to create healthy dishes to share? Joining or forming a book club that focuses on spiritual and self-empowerment books is another way to strengthen your resolve, reach out to others, and share skills. And it's a low-key, monthly commitment that doesn't require anything more than reading, meeting up, and sharing in a discussion. Volunteer as a patient advocate, or help another person who may be struggling. There are so many things we can do to share what we know and put forth positive energy that will come back to us a hundredfold.

▼ ▼ ▼

Hey, beautiful, I can't believe it's time to say good-bye, can you? We've been on a wild ride together, and my hope is that you found it enlightening, supportive, fun, and most of all, helpful. I can tell you that I laughed and cried while working on this book. I put my whole heart and soul into it, and I hope it showed and that you felt it. Maybe you laughed and cried too. Maybe you recognized yourself and learned that you are not alone. Because you're not! We are in this together. It took some courage for me to reveal my story, my mistakes, and my successes in my journey toward wellness. It was a risk I was willing to take because I believe in your power to do the same. *I know you can do it.* I know you can release your inner Glow Warrior.

You have a brand-new set of tools that set you up to thrive and kick sick's ass. If ever you feel lost along the way, come back to this book and use it as your resource. Continue to challenge yourself. Nothing great ever comes from feeling comfortable; there is a better way for you to feel than the way you feel now.

Marianne Williamson says, "We do not heal the past by dwelling there; we heal the past by living fully in the present."[1] This means that every moment you feel yourself drive off course, you have the ability to take a deep breath, connect with yourself, and get back on the right path, in the present moment. Once again, put your hand to your heart and feel it beating—that's you, dear heart. Don't waste a minute.

KICKING SICK *Action Plan Journal*

What follows is a journal to help you start putting everything we've talked about in the book into action in your own life. Each time you do a part of the action plan, make a note of it here. Oh, and pat yourself on the back! Job well done. Check it off the list and make a note of how you felt.

1 REMIND YOURSELF OF YOUR *True Identity*

My favorite mantras

_____

_____

_____

_____

_____

How I felt

_____

_____

_____

_____

2 SET YOURSELF UP FOR *Success*

What I did

How it made me feel

3 SET UP YOUR *A-Team*

How I organized my A-team

Who I added

Who I tossed

How it helped

How I feel now versus then

4 Clean House

What I did

How it changed my mood

5 PRACTICE Self-Care

My new self-care routine

How it improved my daily functioning

How I feel now versus then

What I'm eating

How I feel now that I'm eating well

7 Get Moving

My favorite activities

_____

_____

_____

_____

How it improved my mood and self-image

_____

_____

_____

_____

_____

Length of workout

_____

_____

_____

_____

How I feel now that I work out regularly versus how I felt then when I wasn't

_____

_____

_____

_____

My favorite wellness workers

Improvements in myself and my health

9 CONNECT WITH YOUR *Higher Self*

My spiritual practices

My best times for spiritual practice

New things I am adding to my routine

How I feel after I practice them

10 CREATE A TRIBE YOU *Love*

The important people to me are

_____

_____

_____

_____

I let them know I cherish them by

_____

_____

_____

_____

What I need from them that will help us stay connected

_____

_____

_____

_____

11 BE YOUR OWN *Best Friend*

My positive self-talk

_____

_____

_____

_____

_____

_____

_____

My strategy for dealing with negative self-talk

_____

_____

_____

_____

_____

_____

_____

12 SHARE THE *Glow*

What I am most excited about on my wellness journey

_____

_____

_____

_____

_____

Ways I can share my enthusiasm

_____

_____

_____

_____

_____

✓ More

Did any new self-care ideas come to mind after you read chapter 2? Want to record your "Dream Doc" list from chapter 4, or write down the names and contact information for your own A-team? Are there any new fitness activities you'd like to try or an exercise mantra you'd like to road test after reading chapter 7? Need a place to jot down the new-and-improved beliefs you've shifted into after reading chapter 8? Here are some Kicking Sick journal pages to make your own. Dream big!

Notes

Chapter 1
What's Amy Got to Do With It?

1 Centers for Disease Control and Prevention, "Chronic Disease Overview." Available online at cdc.gov/chronicdisease/overview/index.htm, accessed June 7, 2016.

Chapter 3
Self-Care Is Health Care

1 Oprah Winfrey Network, "Brené Brown: 3 Things You Can Do to Stop a Shame Spiral" (October 6, 2013). Available online at youtube.com/watch?v=TdtabNt4S7E, accessed June 7, 2016.

2 Jeremy Appleton, "Lavender Oil for Anxiety and Depression: Review of the Literature on the Safety and Efficacy of Lavender," *Natural Medicine Journal* 4, no. 2 (February 2012). Available online at naturalmedicinejournal.com/journal/2012-02/lavender-oil-anxiety-and-depression-0.

3 P. J. Murphy and S. S. Campbell, "Nighttime Drop in Body Temperature: A Physiological Trigger for Sleep Onset?" *Sleep* 20, no. 7 (July 1997), 505–11. Abstract available online at ncbi.nlm.nih.gov/pubmed/9322266.

4 "How Much Sleep Do We Really Need?" Available online from the National Sleep Foundation at sleepfoundation.org/how-sleep-works/how-much-sleep-do-we-really-need/page/02.

Chapter 5
Wellness Work 101

1 Emotional Deprivation in Infancy: Study by René A. Spitz 1952. Available online at fullreels.com/en/video/VvdOe10vrs4/Emotional-Deprivation-in-Infancy-Study-by-Rene-A-Spitz-1952.

2 Harry F. Harlow, "Love in Infant Monkeys," *Scientific American* 200 (June 1959): 68, 70, 72–73, 74. Transcript available online at pages.uoregon.edu/adoption/archive/HarlowLIM.htm.

3 Ashley M. Smith, Timothy J. Loving, Erin E. Crockett, and Lorne Campbell, "What's Closeness Got to Do with It? Men's and Women's Cortisol Responses When Providing and Receiving Support," *Psychosomatic Medicine* 71, no. 8 (October 2009): 843–51. Abstract available online at journals.lww.com/psychosomaticmedicine/Abstract/2009/10000/What's Closeness Got to Do withItMensand.6.aspx.

Chapter 7
Movin' On Up

1 Mark Hyman, "You Can't Exercise Your Way Out of a Bad Diet, But Here are 7 Reasons Why Exercise is Still Important" (September 13, 2015), drhyman.com/blog/2015/09/11/you-cant-exercise-your-way-out-of-a-bad-diet-but-here-are-7-reasons-why-exercise-is-still-important.

2 Belinda L. Needham et al., "Trajectories of Change in Obesity and Symptoms of Depression: The CARDIA Study," *American Journal of Public Health* 100, no. 6 (June 2010):1040–6. Abstract available online at ajph.aphapublications.org/doi/abs/10.2105/AJPH.2009.172809. See also: J. A. Blumenthal et al., "Effects of Exercise Training on Older Patients with Major Depression," *Archives of Internal Medicine* 159, no. 19 (October 25, 1999): 2349–56. Abstract available online at ncbi.nlm.nih.gov/pubmed/10547175.

3 C.D. Rethorst and M. H. Trivedi, "Evidence-Based Recommendations for the Prescription of Exercise for Major Depressive Disorder," *Journal of Psychiatric Practice* 19, no. 3 (May 2013): 204–12. doi: 10.1097/01.pra.0000430504.16952.3e.

4 Richard Louv, *The Nature Principle: Reconnecting with Life in a Virtual Age.* (New York: Algonquin Books, 2011).

5 J. Thompson Coon et al., "Does Participating in Physical Activity in Outdoor Natural Environments Have a Greater Effect on Physical and Mental Wellbeing than Physical Activity Indoors? A Systematic Review," *Environmental Science and Technology* (February 3, 2011). doi: 10.1021/es102947t.

Chapter 10
Smile! You're a Glow Warrior!

1 Marianne Williamson, "The Time That Matters Most," *The Oprah Magazine* (July 2000). Available online at oprah.com/spirit/Marianne-Williamson-The-Time-That-Matters-Most, accessed June 7, 2016.

Resources

For more information about me, and what I do, please visit amykurtz.com and kickingsick.com.

Here are some of my favorite places to go and products to use—they enrich and enhance my life, so I hope you find some gems here too.

Websites

DRHYMAN.COM Mark Hyman's official website

DRJOELEVANS.COM and CENTERFORWOMENSHEALTH.COM Joel Evans' official website and his women's health center website

DTXNYC.COM DTX Cellular Evolution. Specializes in colon hydrotherapy and infrared sauna; Cindy Suarez's official website

ELENABROWER.COM Elena Brower's official website; includes her audio meditation course

EVOLVINGWELL.COM and GLUTENFREESCHOOL.COM Jennifer Fugo's official website and her gluten-free cooking school

GABBYB.TV Gabrielle Bernstein's official website

HANDELGROUP.COM The Handel Group's official website

HOWYOUGLOW.COM Tara Sowlaty and Jessie Groveman's official website

JESSICAORTNER.COM Jessica Ortner's official website

KRISCARR.COM Kris Carr's official website

TERRICOLE.COM Terri Cole's official website

THOMKNOLES.COM Thom Knoles's official website

ULTRAWELLNESSCENTER.COM The UltraWellness Center of Lenox, Massachusetts, official website

YOGAGLO.COM Yoga instruction and information

ZIVAMEDITATION.COM Meditation instruction and information

Reading

BERNSTEIN, GABRIELLE. *Spirit Junkie: A Radical Road to Self-Love and Miracles.* Harmony, 2011.

BERNSTEIN, GABRIELLE. *Miracles Now: 108 Life-Changing Tools for Less Stress, More Flow, and Finding Your True Purpose.* Hay House, 2014.

BERNSTEIN, GABRIELLE. *The Universe Has Your Back: Transform Fear to Faith.* Hay House, 2016.

BLAND, JEFFREY S. *The Disease Delusion.* HarperWave, an imprint of Harper Collins, 2014.

BLUM, SUSAN. *The Immune System Recovery Plan.* Scribner, 2013.

BRACH, TARA. *Radical Acceptance: Embracing Your Life with the Heart of a Buddha.* Bantam Books, 2003.

BRACH, TARA. *Radical Acceptance.* Bantam, 2004.

BROWER, ELENA and ERICA JAGO. *Art of Attention: A Yoga Practice Workbook for Movement as Meditation.* Sounds True, 2016.

CAMPBELL, T. COLIN and THOMAS M. CAMPBELL II. *The China Study.* BenBella Books, 2005.

CARR, KRIS. *Crazy Sexy Cancer Survivor: More Rebellion and Fire for Your Healing Journey.* Skirt!, 2008.

CARR, KRIS. *Crazy Sexy Cancer Tips.* Skirt!, 2007.

CARR, KRIS. *Crazy Sexy Diet: Eat Your Veggies, Ignite Your Spark, and Live Life Like You Mean It!* Skirt!, 2011.

HAY, LOUISE. *I Can Do It—How to Use Affirmations to Change Your Life.* Hay House, 2003.

HAY, LOUISE. *You Can Heal Your Life.* Hay House, 1987.

HYMAN, MARK. *The Blood Sugar Solution: The Ultra Healthy Program for Losing Weight, Preventing Disease, and Feeling Great Now!* Little, Brown, and Company, 2012.

HYMAN, MARK. *Eat Fat, Get Thin: Why the Fat We Eat is the Key to Sustained Weight Loss and Vibrant Health.* Little, Brown, and Company, 2016.

HYMAN, MARK. *The Ultramind Solution: The Simple Way to Defeat Depression, Overcome Anxiety, and Sharpen Your Mind.* Scribner, 2008.

LAPORTE, DANIELLE. *The Desire Map: A Guide to Creating Goals with Soul.* Sounds True, 2014.

LIPMAN, FRANK and DANIELLE CARO. *The New Health Rules: Simple Changes to Achieve Whole-Body Wellness.* Artisan, 2015.

NICHTERN, ETHAN. *The Road Home: A Contemporary Exploration of the Buddhist Path.* Audible Studios on Brilliance, 2015.

RUIZ, MIQUEL. *The Four Agreements: A Practical Guide to Personal Freedom.* Amber-Allen, 1997.

TOLLE, ECKHART. *The Power of Now.* Namaste Publishing, 2007.

Products

Here are a few of my favorite things that help my self-care practice.

VITAMIX BLENDER high-end, top-of-the-line blender that will last a lifetime, vitamix.com

BREVILLE JUICER affordable, dependable juicer, brevilleusa.com

DŌTERRA ESSENTIAL OILS doterra.com/US/en/

YOUNG LIVING ESSENTIAL OILS youngliving.com

CHANSON EDEN COUNTERTOP WATER IONIZER chansonalkalinewater.com/cart/water-ionizers/ionizers/chanson-eden-water-ionizer-counter-top.html

SUSOSU HYDRIONATOR PORTABLE WATER BOTTLE IONIZER available at Amazon and other online and retail stores

PANGEA ORGANICS natural skin and body care products, pangeaorganics.com

CONSCIOUS COCONUT high-quality coconut oil, consciouscoconut.com

Art Credits

Chapter 1

1 Paper background, © Picsfive, shutterstock.com

6 Photos of young Amy, by Barbara Kurtz

7 Photos of Amy at her sister's wedding, by Tyler Boye Photography

8 Photo of Amy in hospital, by Danny Rosensweig

9 Photos of Amy getting tests, by Danny Rosensweig

14 Photo of Kaitlyn Lennon, by Darren Ornitz

15 Photo of Tara Sowlaty, by Emily Knecht

15 Photo of Jennifer Fugo, © Chris Plentus Photography

17 Arrow icon, heart icon, star icon, © Seohwa Kim, shutterstock.com

Chapter 2

27 Photo of Elena Brower, by Pete Longworth

Chapter 3

33 Photo of Kris Carr, © Bill Miles

43 Tapping drawing, © artsandra, shutterstock.com

Chapter 4

64 Checkmark icon, © Irmak Akcadogan, shutterstock.com

Chapter 5

75 Photo of Michael Cindrich, by Deborah Kleinman-Cindrich, DC

79 Photo of Cindy Suarez, by Vadin Lum You

Chapter 6

91 Food plate, © Sudowoodo, shutterstock.com

97 Photo of Gerard Mullin, by Keith Weller/Johns Hopkins Medicine

Chapter 7

Chapter 8

Chapter 9

Acknowledgments

Writing this book has been a labor of love. I would like to acknowledge the following people who were instrumental in making this book a reality.

Sounds True: Thank you to everyone involved for believing in this book and making my dream come true. Tami Simon, thank you for founding Sounds True and for the important work Sounds True puts out in the world. Jennifer Brown, thank you for championing this project from the very beginning and for understanding and believing it was as needed as I did. Amy Rost, my amazing editor: There aren't enough thank yous! Thank you for holding my hand and cheering me on—your support has meant more to me than you know. You have taught me so much. Thank you for your attention to detail and your consistent guidance. Your inspiring quotes on my wall aren't moving any time soon! Leslie Brown, thank you for getting me to the finish line! Brian Galvin, thank you for your excitement, enthusiasm, and your pure heart. Thank you to everyone at Sounds True. I am deeply grateful.

All of the contributors who are a part of this book: Your insights and knowledge have paved the path to my healing. Thank you for your wisdom. Thank you from the deepest part of my heart for sharing it with everyone who will read this book.

To the Glow Warriors: Thank you for sharing your stories throughout the pages of this book with grace, honesty, and courage. You inspire me.

Carol Mann, thank you for helping me make this a reality from the ground up, and for believing in what *Kicking Sick* could be since the very beginning! I'm forever grateful for your commitment and your guidance.

Karen Kelly, my editor, teacher, and friend: Thank you for being my teammate in this process, for your guidance, and for your support. I am so grateful for you. It's been an honor. Thank you for getting me and "getting it" before there were even words on a page, and helping me turn *Kicking Sick* into a book! You are the best.

Mom and Dad, there are no words to truly tell you how much your support on this journey has meant to me. Thank you for everything. Thank you for your unlimited love, strength, and consistency. Thank you for trusting me to trust my gut even if it took us out of our comfort zone! I am so grateful for you. I love you endlessly.

Dana and Liza, thank you for teaching me my first life lessons and for always showing me the way.

Danny, thank you for holding the space for me to go for my dream. Your belief in this project and me has been unwavering, and I am forever grateful to you for your love and support. You have taught me more than you can imagine. You have supported and encouraged me in a way that touches my heart so deeply. Thank you.

Elena, thank you for being the lighthouse for me and for showing up for this project in the way that you have. Thank you for continually showing up and believing in this book and me.

Kris, thank you for writing your books and for being brave enough to share your story with the world. You changed my life forever, and lit a spark in me. I am so grateful I found your work. You are magic.

Lauren, thank you for showing me that the dreams we have are completely possible, for your unwavering support, and for your unconditional love. I am forever grateful for you. Thank you for helping me to manifest my dreams.

Mark, thank you for helping me figure out my health challenge and for helping me heal. Thank you for being a part of this project and giving me the honor of having you write the forward for this book. I am truly so grateful that you are a part of my story and for all of your help.

Thank you to every one of my clients for our work together, for all of your inside-out transformations, and for all of the successes we have shared together. Thank you for opening my eyes further to see that this story needed to be told in order to serve others. I am forever thankful to have been by your side cheering you on and for all of the lessons that our work together has taught me.

Index

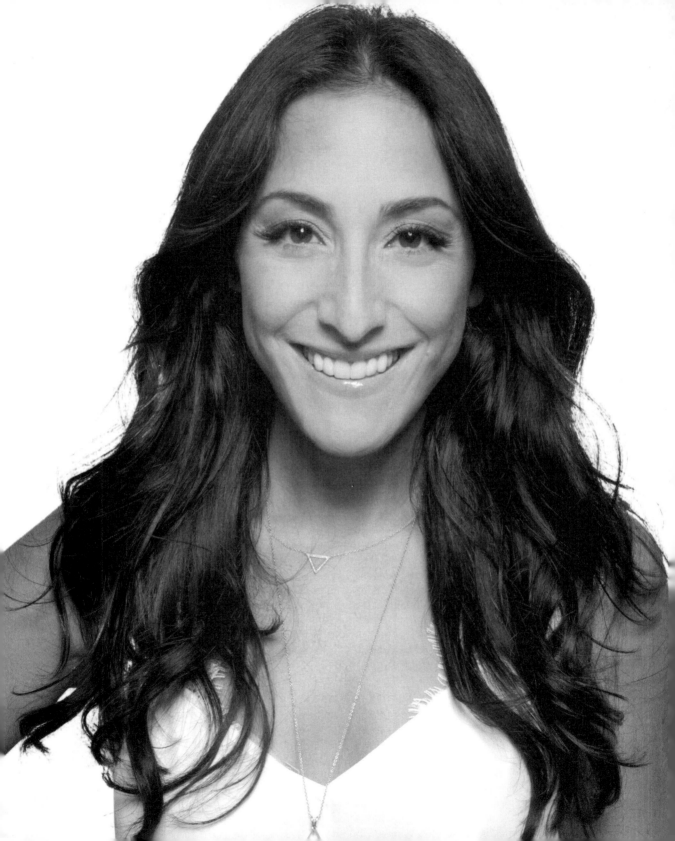

About the Author

AMY KURTZ is a health and wellness expert, teacher, writer, and former full-time patient. She is a board-certified AADP Holistic Health Coach (HHC), with certification from the Institute of Integrative Nutrition in New York City, and a member of the American Association of Drugless Practitioners (AADP). Amy is also a Kane School–certified Pilates trainer (CPT) and a certified Woods Gravity Colon Therapist (WGCT). During her health coach training, she studied more than one hundred dietary theories, innovative coaching methods, and practical lifestyle management techniques with some of the world's top health and wellness experts. Her teachers included Dr. Andrew Weil, Dr. Mark Hyman, and Dr. Deepak Chopra. She has also worked alongside a prominent Functional Medicine doctor in NYC as the health coach for his practice, before embarking on her own.

Amy has radically improved her health, and today she's helping people of all ages live well regardless of their health situation. Many of her clients have acute chronic conditions, and she helps them to stabilize and manage their conditions by providing guidance and helping them create the right team of health care professionals. She also helps clients learn and make self-care regimes a priority, and to become an active participant in their healing journey. She empowers them to embark on their own wellness revolution.

Amy is a regular contributor on popular websites including mindbodygreen.com and yoganonymous.com. She lives in New York City.

For more info on Amy and her universe, check out amykurtz.com.

About Sounds True

Sounds True is a multimedia publisher whose mission is to inspire and support personal transformation and spiritual awakening. Founded in 1985 and located in Boulder, Colorado, we work with many of the leading spiritual teachers, thinkers, healers, and visionary artists of our time. We strive with every title to preserve the essential "living wisdom" of the author or artist. It is our goal to create products that not only provide information to a reader or listener, but that also embody the quality of a wisdom transmission.

For those seeking genuine transformation, Sounds True is your trusted partner. At SoundsTrue.com you will find a wealth of free resources to support your journey, including exclusive weekly audio interviews, free downloads, interactive learning tools, and other special savings on all our titles.

To learn more, please visit SoundsTrue.com/freegifts or call us toll-free at 800.333.9185.

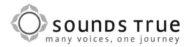

SOUNDS TRUE
many voices, one journey